WONDERFULLY MADE

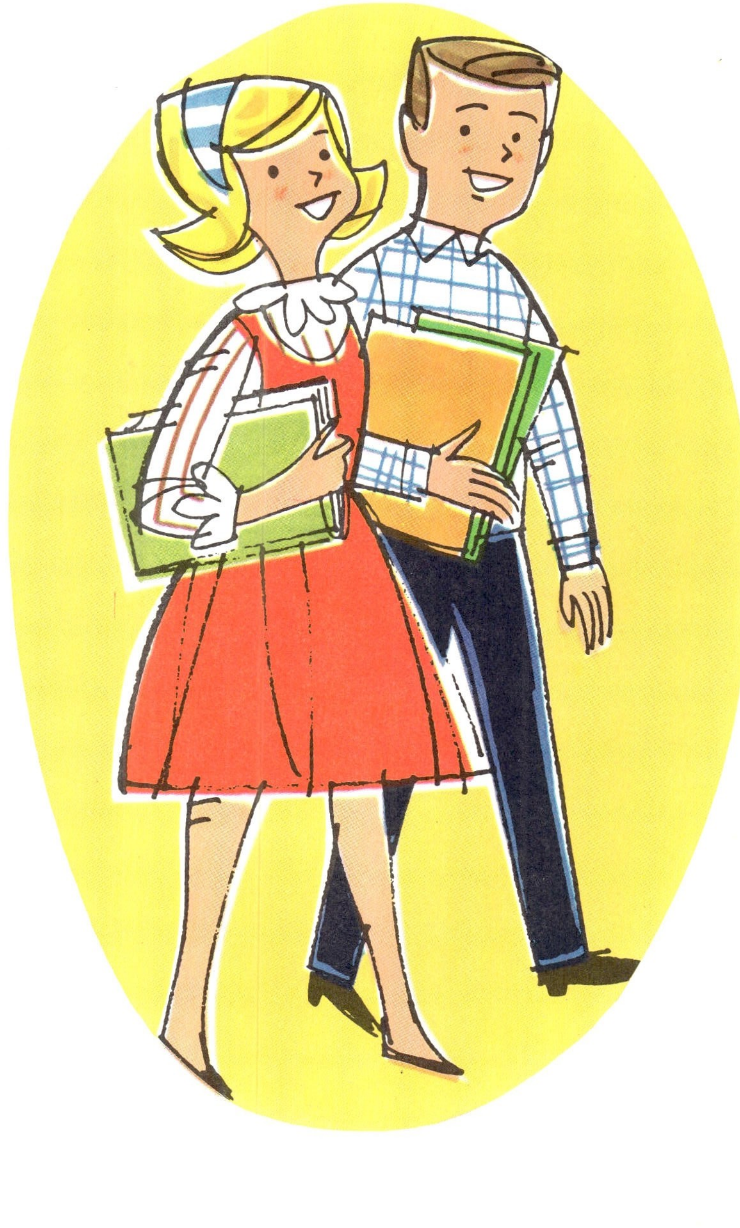

TEXT/By Ruth Hummel

EDITOR/W. J. Fields

ART / Concordia Films

Concordia Publishing House
Saint Louis London

"What does it mean to grow up?" Bob asked himself. He was just your age and as active as you are. Studying his lessons, meeting his friends, and working on his hobbies seemed to take every minute of his day. Yet he couldn't help thinking about growing up.

"What will growing up mean for me?" he wondered.

All boys and girls your age want to know about growing up. They plan what they will be. They imagine doing exciting things when they are on their own. They are puzzled about what the future will be like. They don't want their dreams to turn out to be fairy tales. They want the facts, the truth.

FULL OF LIFE

ALIVE AND GROWING

Your body has been growing steadily ever since you could walk. Each part of your body is growing—the bones, the muscles, and the nerves. The bones in your body grow longer and thicker, and the flesh on your bones grows to fit. The different parts of your body grow at exactly the right rate of speed, so that growth remains regular.

Many changes take place while your body is growing larger and heavier. One of these changes is the hardening of the bones. A baby has many bones that are soft in places. These soft parts are not really bone yet and are called *cartilage.* This cartilage is like the gristle in meat, which you know is tough and chewy.

"Be careful of the soft spots on Baby's head!" If you've been around a young baby, you have probably heard this warning. Besides the two soft spots on the head, other bones in the body are also partly soft cartilage when we are born. Growing takes place only in the cartilage at the ends of these bones. As the body grows to its full height, the cartilage gradually hardens until all is bone. Then growth stops.

Concordia Publishing House, St. Louis, Missouri
Concordia Publishing House Ltd., London, E. C. 1

Library of Congress Catalog Card No. 67-24878
MANUFACTURED IN THE UNITED STATES OF AMERICA

This happens sometime between the ages of 16 and 20. Though each person has his own growth schedule, we can speak of averages. If you are a girl, you will probably reach your full height a few years earlier than the boys your age.

GROWING UP

Some of the most important changes that take place during your growing years occur in your thinking and acting. Wouldn't it be strange to see people your size acting and thinking like small children? It's a good thing your growing takes place over many years. You need this time to learn to think and act as an adult by the time your body grows up. Each day is full of so many things to do, to work out, and to play at.

"You're sure on the go today," John's mother said. John had rushed in from school a few minutes earlier. Now he was leaving again. He had taken only a minute to change into his

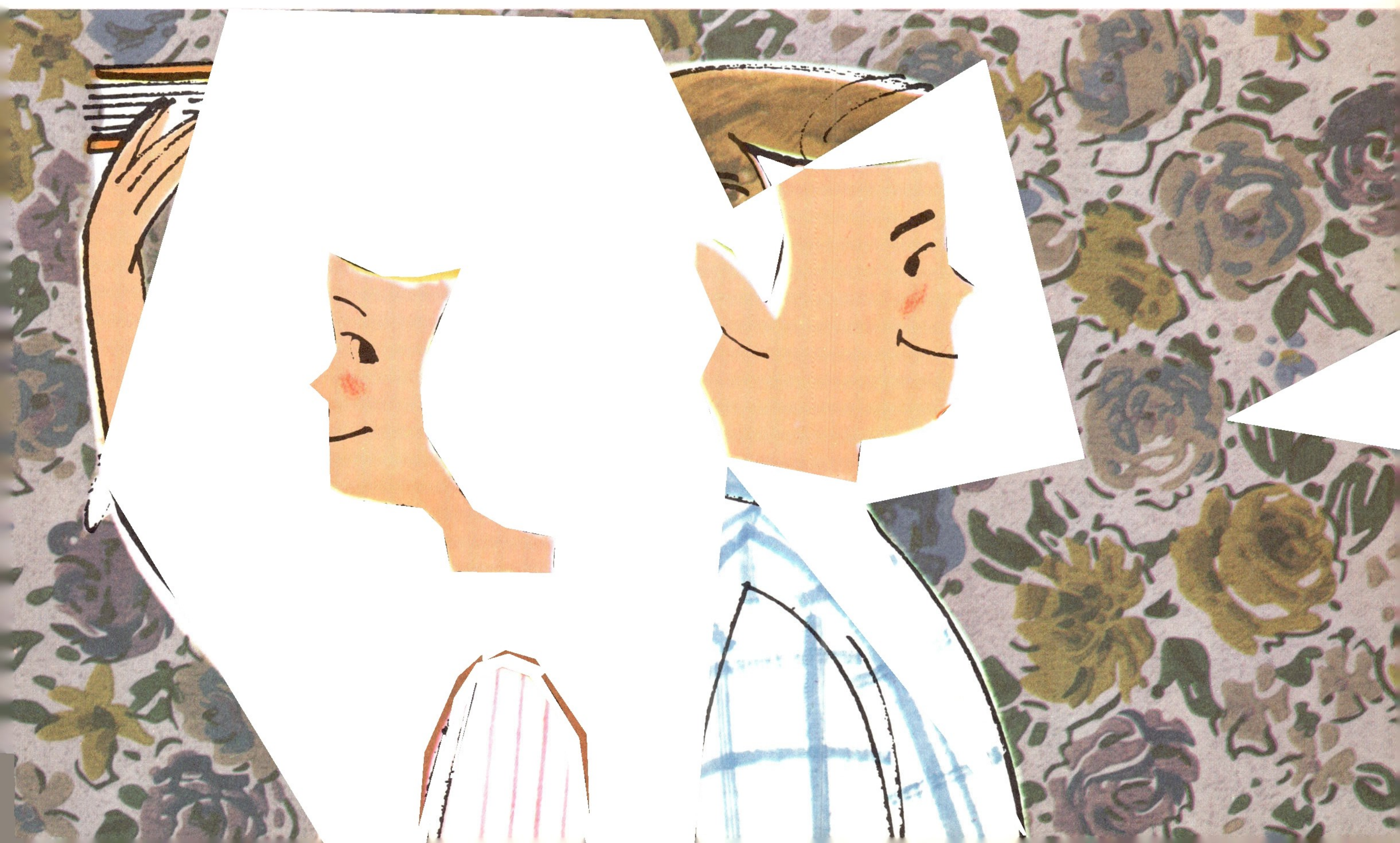

jeans and old red sweater. Another minute to down a glass of milk and a sandwich. Now with ball, bat, and glove he headed for the door.

"I'll be back in time for my paper route," he called. Then the door banged behind him.

John has a full life. An exciting ball game, his own job, then home for supper with his family. After that, homework and a little work on his rock collection before bed.

John is too busy to think about what he is learning in these activities. But by solving his problems and correcting his mistakes he is becoming more grown up each day.

He is sticking to his job and proud that people can rely on him. He is realizing how important fair play is in getting along with others. He is learning more about himself—what he can do, what he likes, and what people like about him. Although he is learning to take care of himself better each day, he still ap-

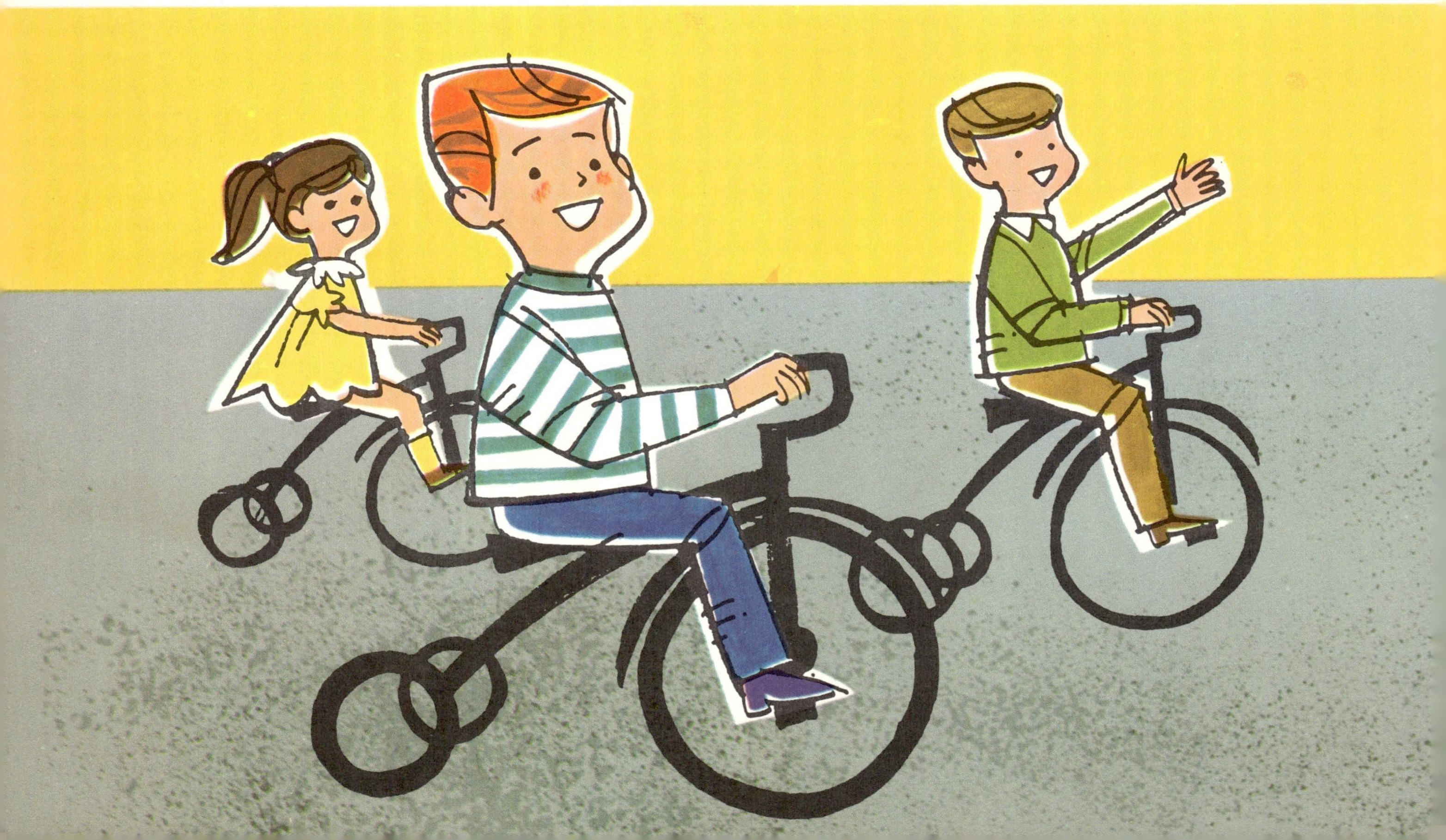

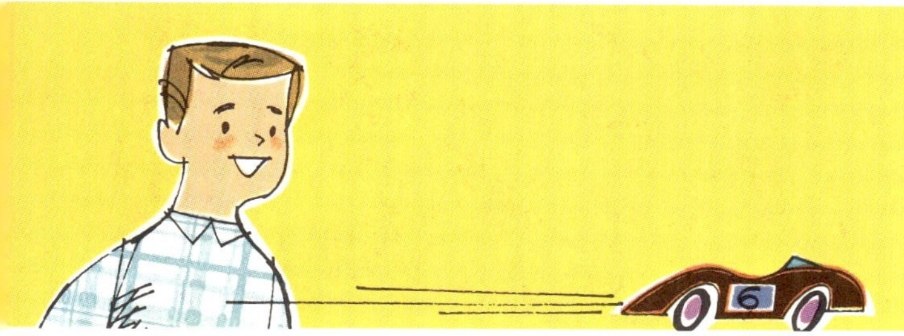

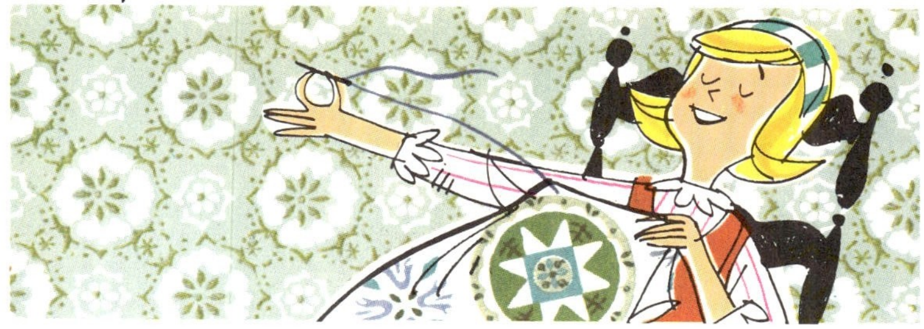

preciates the understanding and love he gets from his family. John is on the way to becoming an adult.

GROWING AS BOYS AND GIRLS

Growing up also brings changes in the feelings boys and girls have about each other. When you were a baby, you didn't care whether you played with boys or girls. Very small children can't even use "he" and "she" correctly. Even kindergarten children play "house" together and are interested in many of the same toys.

Then the time comes when boys' and girls' interests begin to differ. Boys become interested in the things that are called "masculine." They picture themselves as the men they would like to be. They are interested in joining clubs with other boys their age.

A girl becomes interested in "feminine" things. When she looks at women, she sees herself as she will be someday. She and her friends are busy doing and learning the things that women do. She considers boys' games too noisy and rough but begins to have more interest in boys as she nears her teens.

Everyone, though, has his own individual interests. Otherwise life would become very dull. We hear of 4-H girls who raise champion cattle and of boys who win cooking awards. There is no reason for not following our own interests, even if they are slightly different from those of other members of our sex.

Then too, common interests such as playing in a band or orchestra can draw boys and girls together. Going to school together each day affords them many opportunities to get along together. Parties give them a chance to practice the good manners they have learned.

The boy-girl feelings you now have will probably change in

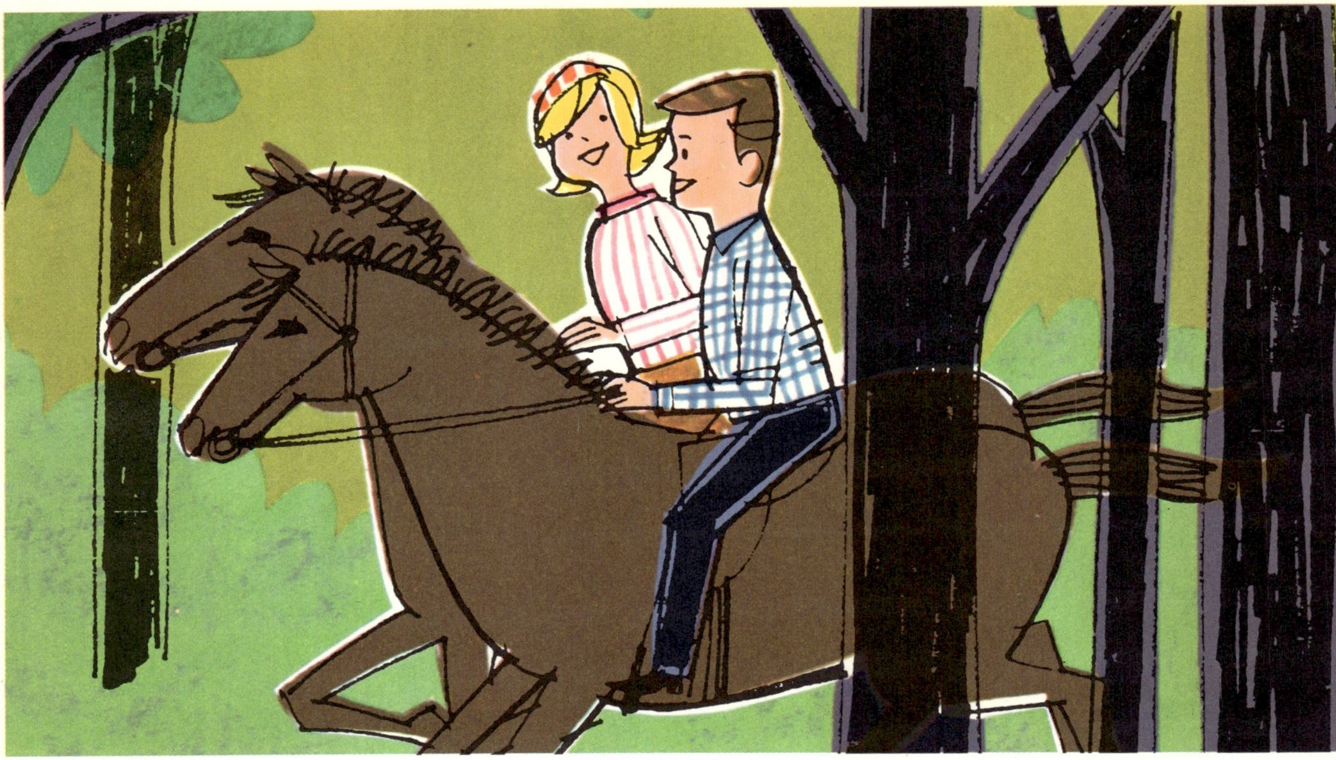

the next few years. During the teen-age years boys and girls find each other far more interesting. You, too, will soon arrive at that stage in life.

WHY BOYS AND GIRLS

Growing up will bring many more changes. Many of them will depend on whether you are growing up to be a man or a woman, for boys and girls develop differently from one another.

Have you ever wondered just why people were made of two sexes?

The answer to this question goes back to God, from whom all life comes.

You share life with countless other creatures of God—plants, animals, and people. God has created many kinds of living things for the world. Each kind is different. Each has been made to carry out its own task. Each has its own reason for being alive.

God wants this life to continue on the earth. He gave to

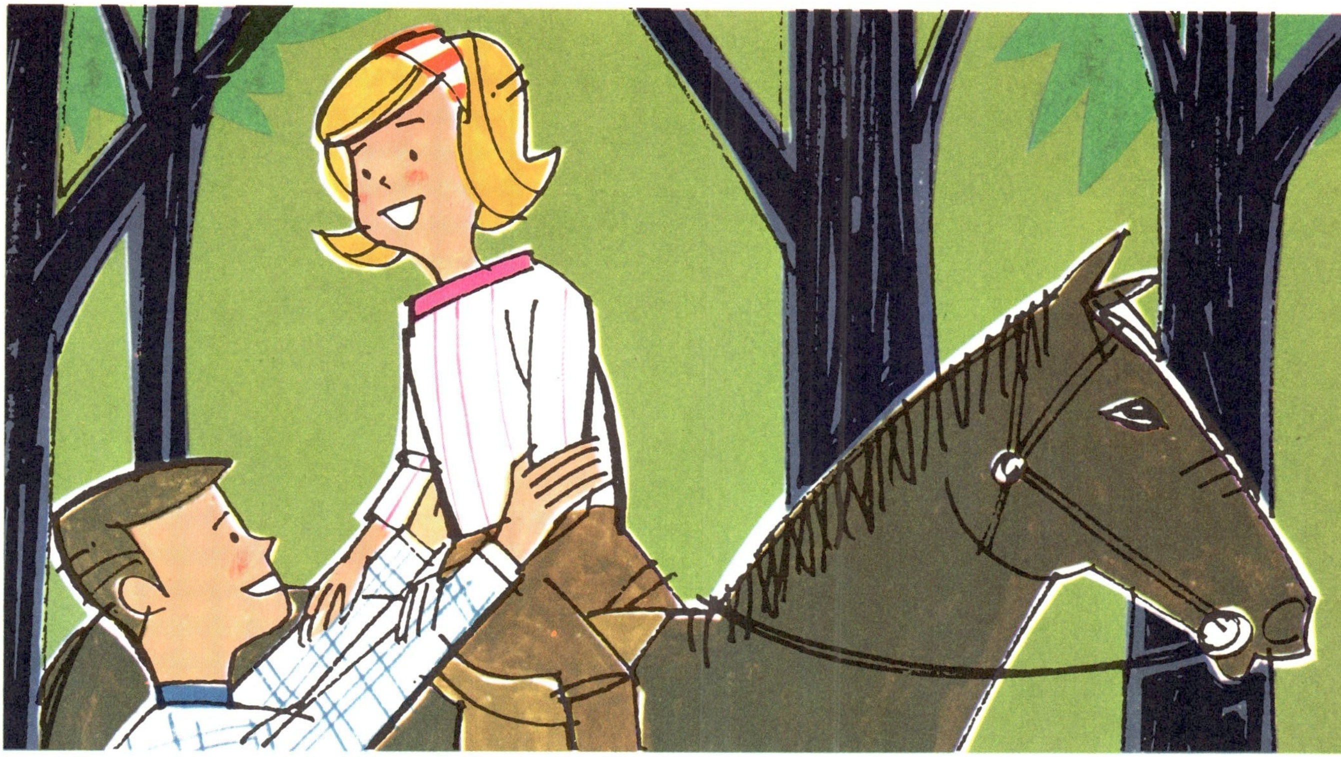

plants, animals, and people the power to pass life on to new beings who will live after them.

Dogs do not have kittens. Pumpkin vines never grow from apple seeds. Each creature's "babies" are like itself. So each type of life goes on.

To start new life, most animals were made either male or female. People, also, are of two sexes. It takes both a father and a mother to bring babies into the world. Each plays a different part, yet both are necessary.

People are more than animals. God loved them in a special way. And as He loved them, so He means for them to love one another. He wants them to be good for one another and to be concerned about one another's well-being. This love is not the "mushy" love you see in the movies or on television. It's the kind of love that Jesus Christ had for people—the kind of love that is always trying to help people and to make their lives better. That really is why God has given us life, our bodies, our abilities, that with them we can make the lives of other people better and happier.

"This birdhouse looked much better last week," George's father said.

George looked surprised. "What do you mean, Dad?" he asked. "We didn't even start making it until yesterday."

George's father laughed. "It was in my mind last week already," he explained. "I could close my eyes and see just how I wanted it to look. But I'm afraid it hasn't turned out that well."

GOD CREATED YOU

Did you ever wonder where you were before your life started? You, too, were first in Someone's mind. Before people existed, God thought of them. He planned how He would give them life. He made them of two sexes, male and female, so they would be able to pass life on to their children.

Men and women are different from one another. But the differences do not make one better than the other. No one needs to wish to be of the other sex. Both sexes are necessary for God's plan. The world could never get along if all the men, or all the women, "were all transported far beyond the northern sea."

MARRIAGE AND FAMILIES

Men and women were made for each other. When they want to get married and have families, that is pleasing to God. He doesn't want people to be lonely or to live only for themselves. Married people soon learn to think of each other. After years of living together, some can almost read each other's thoughts.

By living together and loving each other, a man and woman become as one person. They are still two, of course. Yet people think of them together. Have you heard people calling their husband or wife "my better half"? Though it is usually said jokingly, it does show something. Marriage unites two

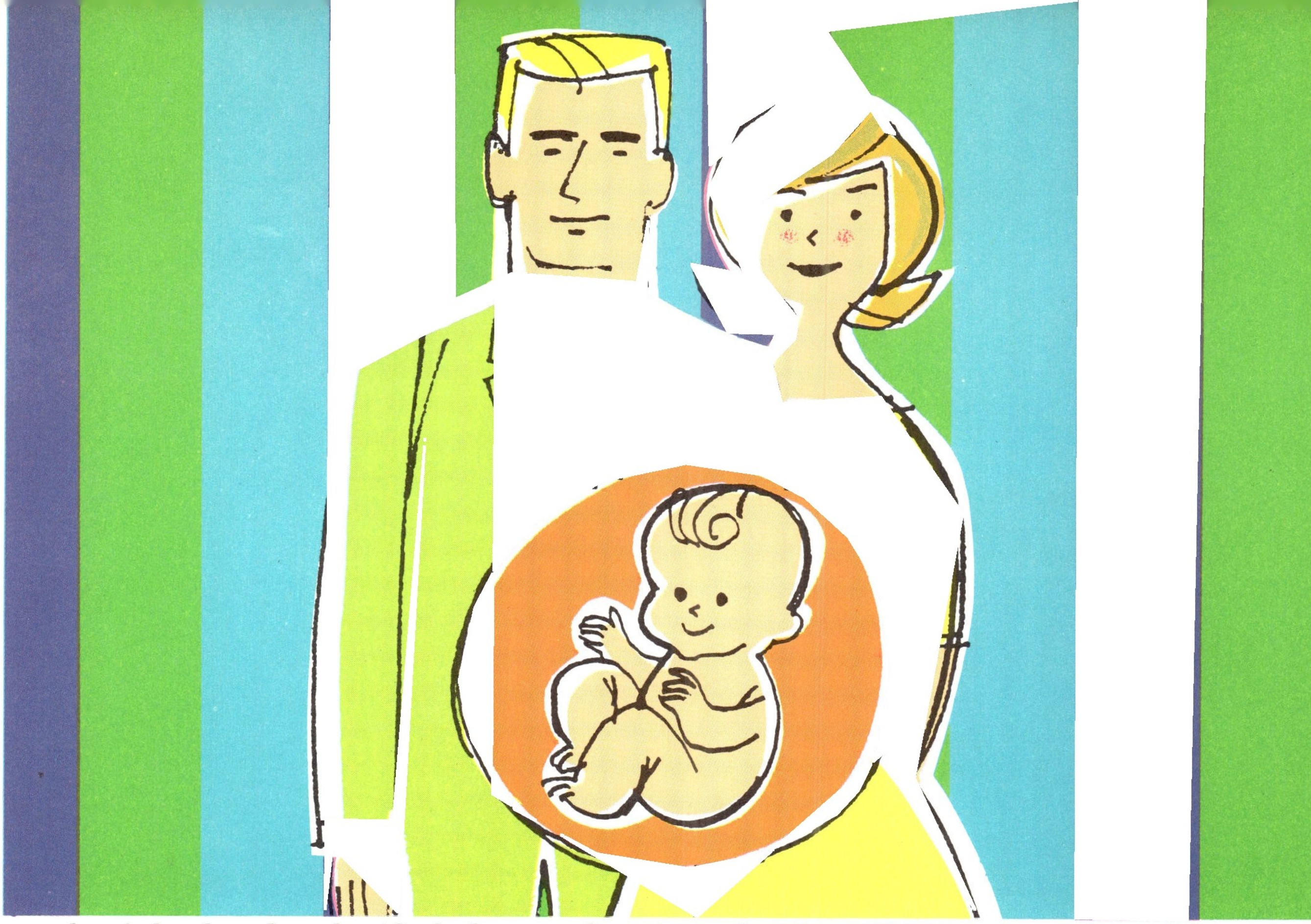

people. A husband and wife feel very close to each other. Deep love and happiness can come from this closeness.

Children are one of the blessings of marriage. They make a marriage into a family. Every baby needs both a father and a mother to receive life. Each one needs a family in which to grow up. Mothers are important both to their boys and to their girls. Fathers can help their sons learn to be men and their daughters grow into women. It is difficult for one person both to support and to care for the child. When one parent has died or is absent for some other reason, relatives and friends sometimes help take their place.

God put you into your family. Your family group is very special for you. It may be large or small. It may include brothers or sisters, one or both parents, or even other relatives. These are the people you know best. Your family is the place where you really "belong."

Everyone in your family is important. It is easy to see how useful your mother or father is. And you have value too. You help make your family a happy one. Even a tiny baby helps do that.

"Our baby sure does," Susan agrees. "He tries to do everything he sees us do, but he never manages it right. He keeps us laughing all day long with his funny tricks."

Families are for living and loving. They can be warm and happy groups, who help one another through times of joy and times of trouble. Families were God's idea. Through persons who love us, God shows His love to us.

WHEN YOU BEGAN

How much do you weigh? Is it 60 pounds, 90 pounds, or somewhere between? Next time you hop on the scale, you will weigh even more. Isn't it hard to believe that you were once a 10-pound baby? But in the beginning you were far smaller than that. When your life began, you were about the size of a grain of sand.

Your body now contains billions and trillions of cells. Yet once you were only one single cell. To form this cell, it took two separate parts—one from your father and one from your mother. Like two raindrops trickling down a window pane, they met and suddenly became only one. Each new life starts this way.

BOY OR GIRL?

The tiny cell that became you had a lot of growing to do. Right from the beginning it was already male or female. Its sex was determined the moment the cells from your parents joined.

The bit of life that came from your mother is called the egg. The part from your father is the *sperm.* The egg cells in a mother are all of one kind, but a father's body makes two different kinds of sperm. If one kind joins an egg, a girl baby will grow. If the sperm happens to be the other kind, the baby will be a boy.

Though there are millions of sperm, there's an equal number of each kind. The baby has an equal chance of being a boy or girl. Think what that means. In this way the number of boys and girls in the world is kept about the same.

When a new baby is on the way to a family, people often try to guess what sex it will be. A family with many boys may wish for a girl, or it may be the other way around. But wishes can't change what was already decided the moment life started.

CHIP OFF THE OLD BLOCK

The members of a family often look like one another.

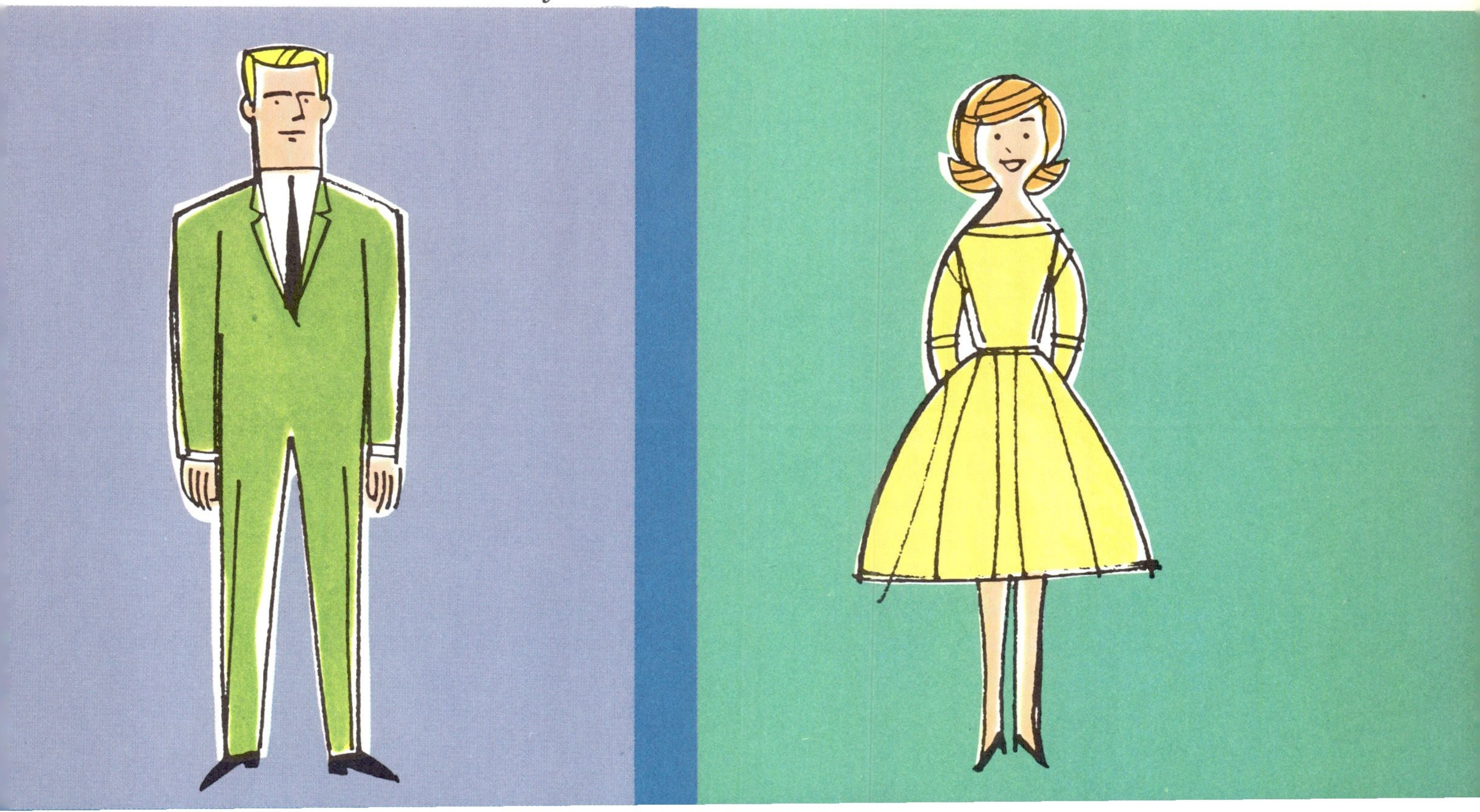

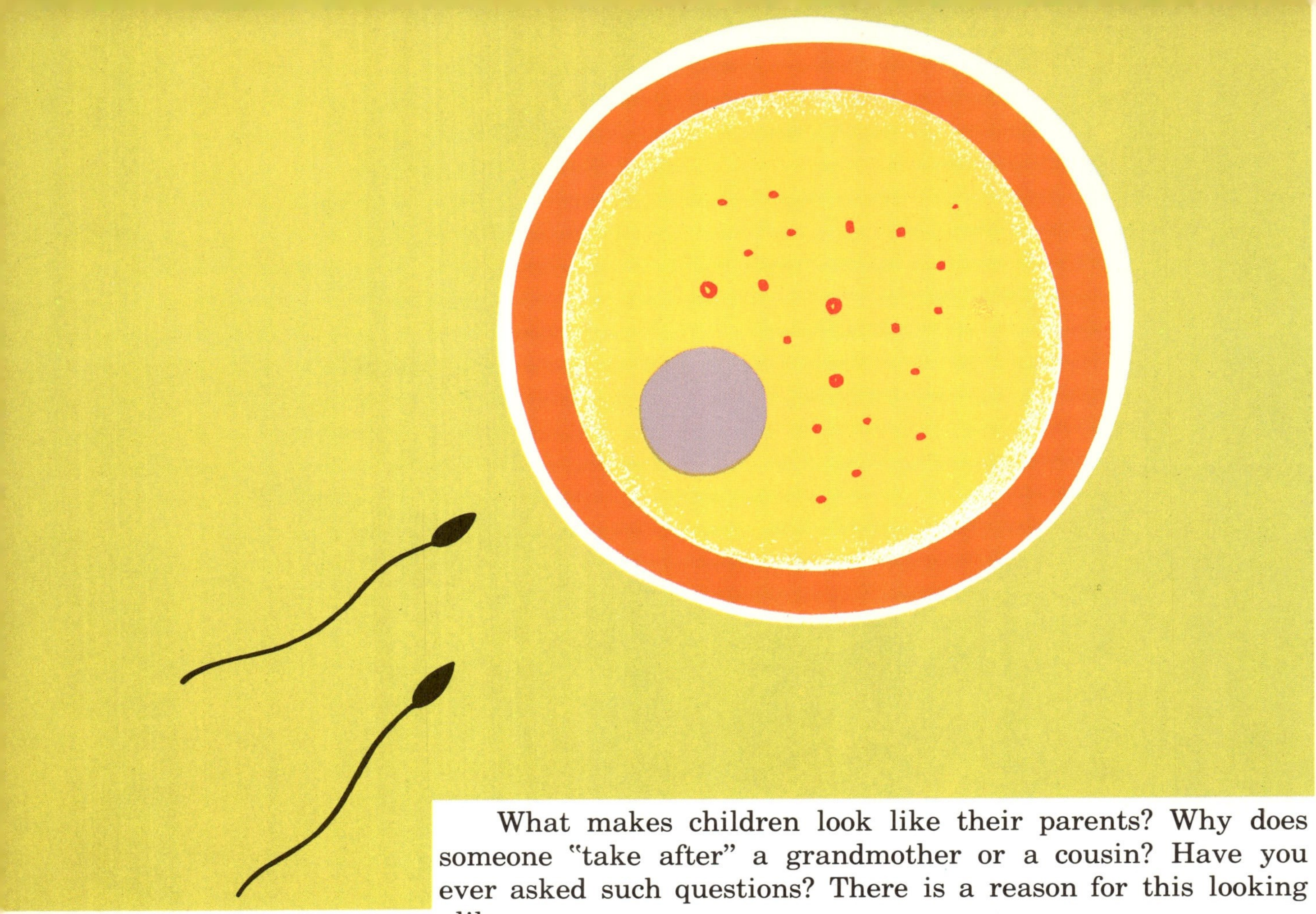

What makes children look like their parents? Why does someone "take after" a grandmother or a cousin? Have you ever asked such questions? There is a reason for this looking alike.

The cell from which you grew was no bigger than a pinpoint. Yet it contained the whole pattern for the person you would become. What color eyes would you have? How tall would you grow? Whom would you look like? Dozens of questions like these were answered in the tiny cell from which you grew. It's hard to imagine how that could be. Yet we know it is true.

Part of this cell came from your father and part from your mother. So it's no wonder that you look something like either or both of them. One may have given you the color of your hair. The other may have given you your tallness.

You may even look like your grandfather or some other relative. Your parents received their *traits,* or characteristics, from your grandparents. Through your parents these features can be passed on to you.

Do you know how many great-great-grandparents you have? Figure it out on this chart.

Parents	2
Grandparents	4
Great-grandparents	8
Great-great-grandparents	?

As the names get longer, the numbers grow larger. Think of all the traits that could have been passed from them to you and your brothers and sisters. Brother Bill may be tall as a bean pole, while everyone calls brother Bob "Shorty." Do you see why this can be?

There are so many different traits among the people of the world. The possible combinations of these traits are so many that you can't begin to count them. There are billions of people in the world. Yet no two are exactly alike. It's all because of one little fact: Each life starts when cells from two different people join.

WHAT ABOUT TWINS?

When a sperm joins an egg cell, usually only one baby grows. Once in a while, however, this *fertilized* egg divides and grows into two babies. These twin babies will have the same traits and be of the same sex. They are called "identical twins" because they are so much alike. Even their mother may have trouble telling them apart at first. But as they grow, each develops in his own way.

Some twins look no more alike than if they were brothers and sisters. These are called, with a word that means brother, "fraternal twins." They grow from two different egg cells. Usually a mother's body makes only one egg at a time. But it sometimes happens that there are two. Then two different sperm can join them. The two babies that grow may have different looks and be of different sexes. So twins, too, are individuals. Each is different from all other people.

Since your father and mother had a part in giving you life, their love for each other has a place in the story of how you began.

They loved each other so much that they decided to marry and to live together. Their wedding day was a happy day for them. Perhaps you have seen their wedding pictures. It was a day they will long remember.

Weddings are joyous events. The bride and groom are happy and excited. The love between husband and wife is deep and satisfying. They are anxious to begin their new life together. Friends and relatives come to wish them well, for there are also problems in making a home. It takes time, work, and patience to make a home that will last.

LOVE BROUGHT YOU TO LIFE

Your parents worked together to build their new life. Each did what he was best suited to do. The work each did was for the other as much as for himself. They helped each other and enjoyed each other's company. Then, because your father and mother loved each other and wanted children, you were born.

God Himself gave people the power to bring children into the world. Creating new life is God's work, but He gave men and women a share in it. Mothers and fathers work together with God when they pass on the gift of life to new beings and when they accept the duty of caring for each new life.

Each parent plays his own part in creating a new life. That is why men and women were made different from each other. Their sex organs, the parts of their bodies that do the work of creating new life, are different.

You have noticed that the bodies of boys and girls are not the same. When boys are born, they have the sex organs that will make sperm. When girls are born, they already have in their bodies partly grown egg cells.

A MOTHER'S SEX ORGANS

Inside every girl's body are two *ovaries* for storing these egg cells. These organs are deep within her body a little lower than the waist. Each one is only as big as an almond; yet thousands of eggs are stored there.

Egg cells are the largest cells in the body, larger than skin cells, muscle cells, or blood cells. Yet they are smaller than the point of a pin. Between the ages of 10 and 14 (sometimes a little earlier, sometimes a little later) work starts in the ovaries. One by one the egg cells begin to change and ripen. After that about once a month an egg cell leaves one or the other ovary.

Near each ovary a hollow tube, called a *Fallopian* tube, opens to receive the egg. While passing through this tube, the egg may meet and unite with a sperm and then continue its journey to the *uterus*. If it does not join a sperm, the egg disintegrates.

The uterus lies between the ovaries and just above the

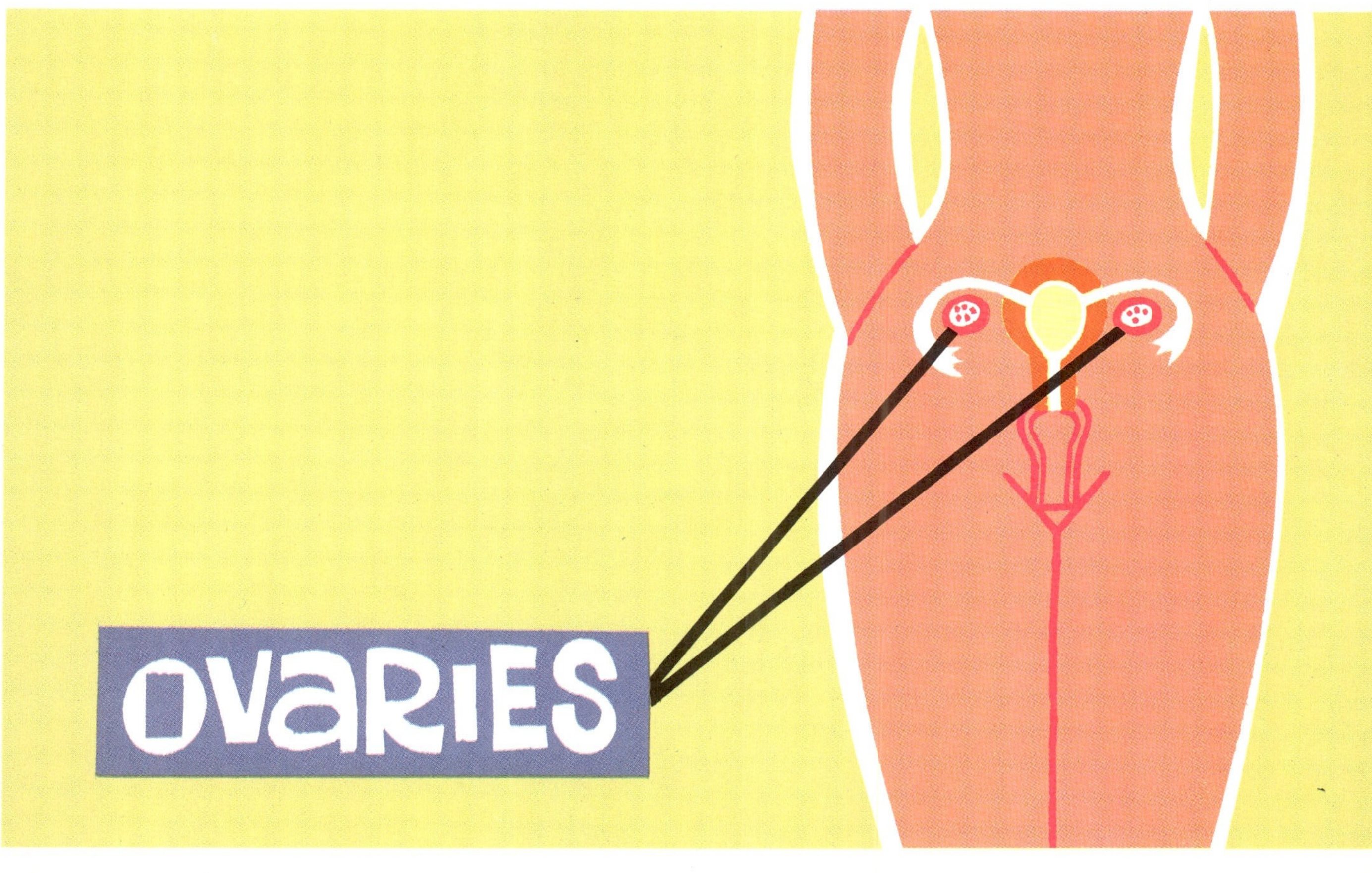

bone that forms a bridge between a girl's legs. It is about the size and shape of a pear. This organ can stretch like a balloon to many times its ordinary size. It is here that a fertilized egg cell grows into a baby.

The uterus is connected to the outside of the body by a narrow passageway. This organ, the *vagina,* opens between the legs. It is covered by folds of skin and flesh called the *vulva.* The opening through which *urine,* or waste water, passes is also within the vulva.

The ovaries, tubes, uterus, vagina, and vulva are the *reproductive* organs of girls and women. All except the vulva are inside the body.

A FATHER'S SEX ORGANS

Most of the male sex organs are on the outside of the body. In two almond-shaped organs called the *testicles,* the sperm ripen. The sperm need a place slightly cooler than body temper-

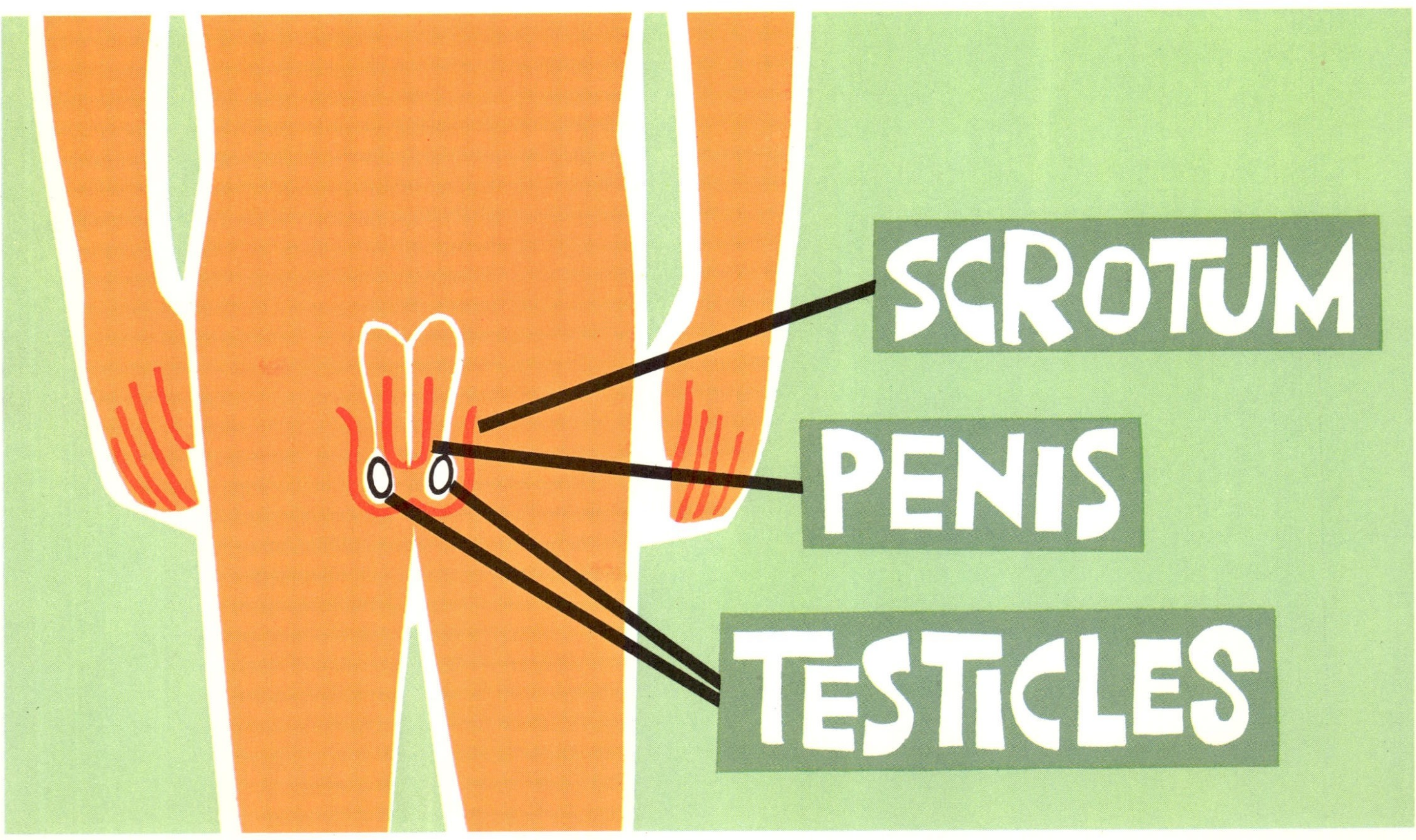

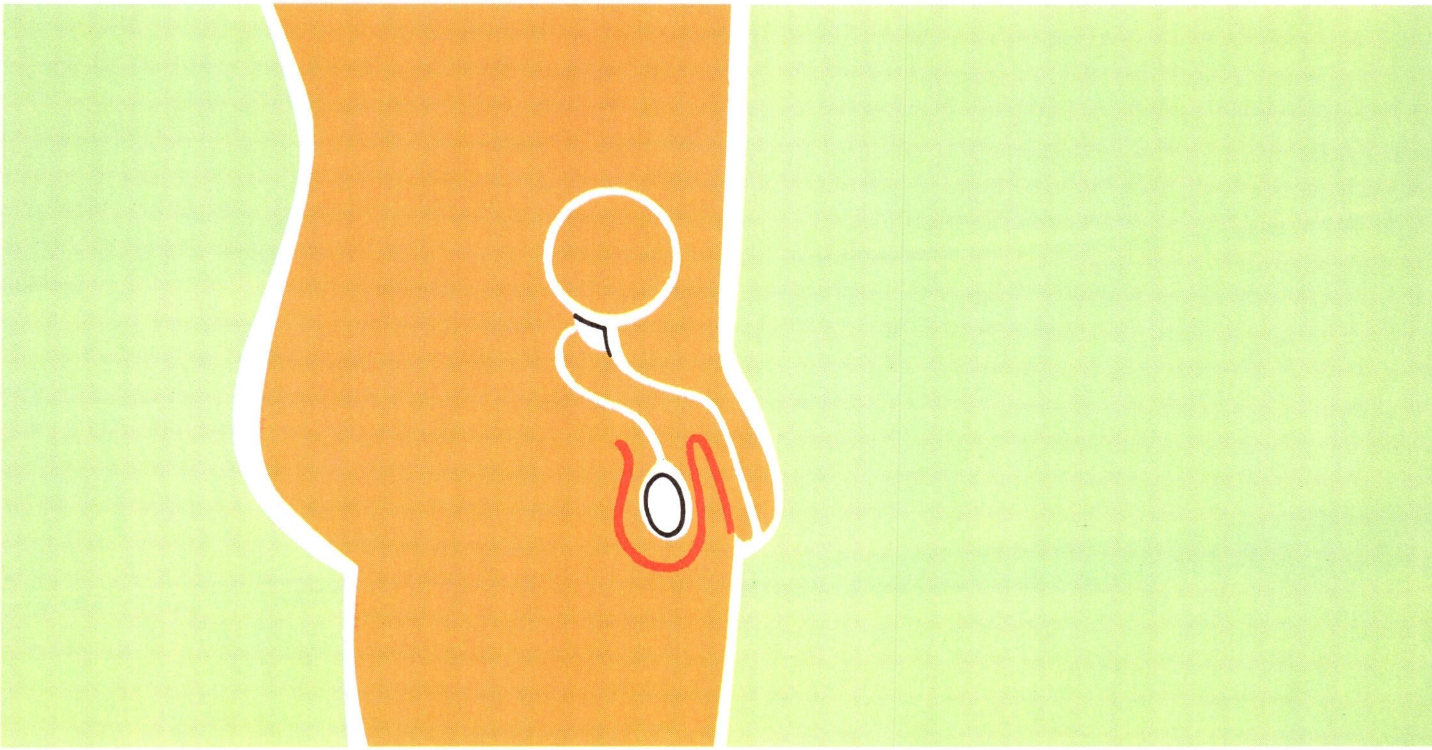

ature. So the testicles are in a sac of skin outside the body. The sac hangs between the legs and is called the *scrotum.*

Sperm are much smaller than egg cells. They look like little tadpoles with long, thin, wiggling tails. In the testicles billions of sperm mature each month. These are stored in a tube something like 20 feet of thin hollow wire curled up in a space smaller than a walnut. This tube becomes thicker and straighter farther up in the body and leads to the outside through the *penis.* This is a finger-shaped organ in front of the scrotum. It is usually soft and spongy.

Between approximately 13 and 15 a boy's body becomes ready to make sperm. It also makes a milky liquid. The sperm can move about quickly in this liquid by whipping their tails. The sperm and the liquid in which they swim is called *semen.* Though the penis is usually soft, at times it becomes firm and erect. Then the semen can pass through it out of the body. Urine also passes out through the penis. Because of a delicate reflex action semen and urine do not normally pass through it at the same time.

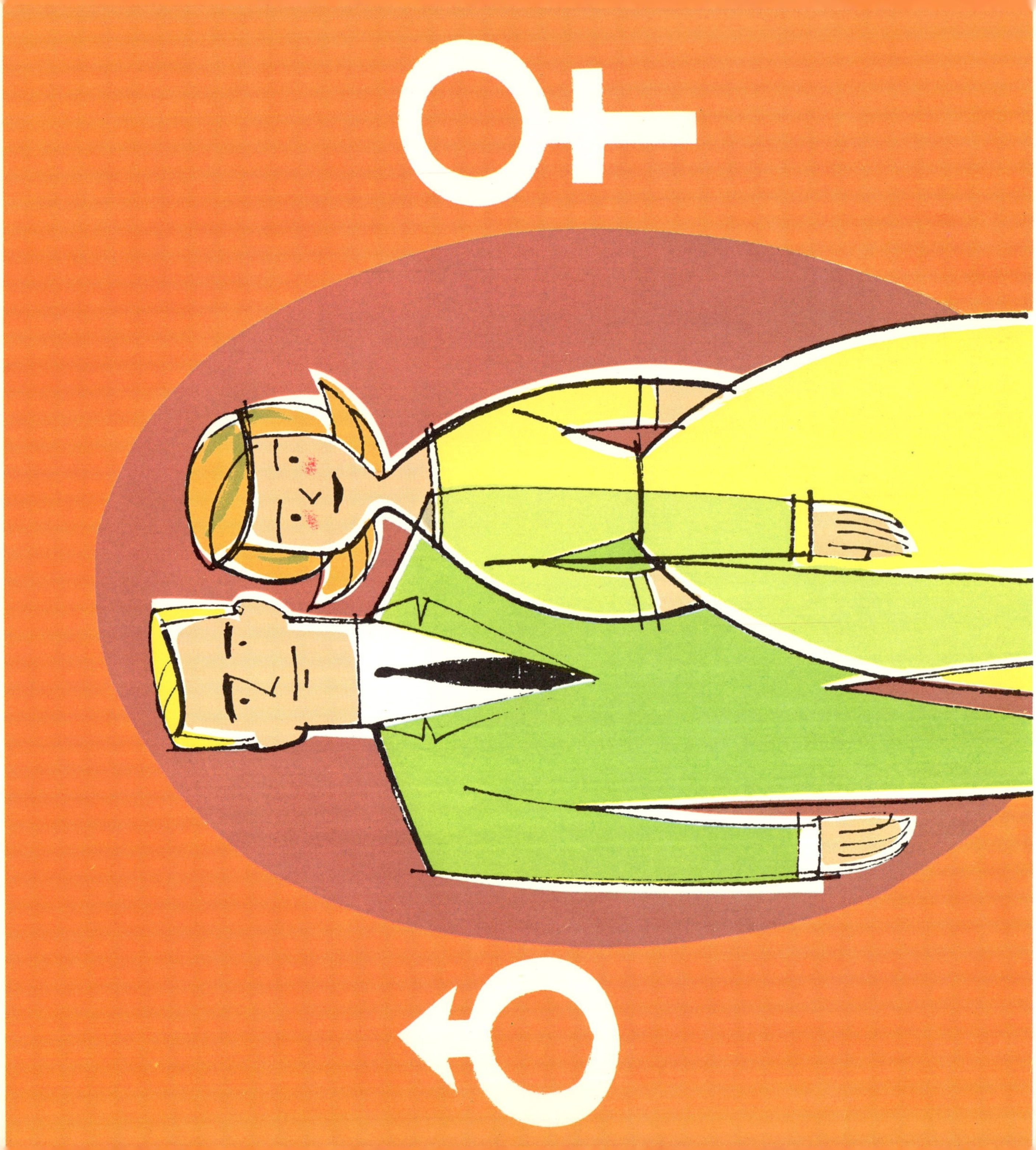

MARRIED LOVE

One of the sperm from the father's body must find and join an egg in the mother's body before a new person can be *conceived,* or start to grow. Here the love of parents comes into the story. In an act of love the father puts the sperm into the mother's body.

Married people show their love in many different ways. Kisses and hugs are among these ways. They also help each other. They share happy times and sad ones. They enjoy just being together. Your parents have their favorite ways of showing love for each other.

At times the love between two married people makes them want to be alone and very close together in an act called sexual intercourse. In this act, sperm leave the father's body and enter the mother's. One of the sperm may unite with an egg cell. The egg cell is then fertilized and begins to grow into a new human being. This is one of God's ways of continuing His creation today. He uses the love of husband and wife to carry on the human race.

A new life doesn't start each time a man and woman have intercourse. An egg cell is in one of the Fallopian tubes only a few days each month, and only then can a baby be conceived. Since it is through intercourse that a baby can begin, God wants only a husband and his wife to make love in this way. Husbands and wives have promised to live together always and to make a home for their children. They as parents will take care of the babies born to them.

This, then, is the story of how your life began. You may have heard the old tale of how the stork brings babies. It wasn't the stork who brought you. The truth is that your parents' love brought you to life.

"So you are moving today," Sam said as he came to watch the movers pack the furniture at Tommy's house into a van. "How come your family decided to buy a new house?"

"This one has gotten too small," Tommy explained. "Our family is growing bigger."

"What's your new house like?" asked Sam.

LIVING IN YOUR FAMILY

"It is a two-story house instead of a ranch style," said Tommy. "Each of us kids will have his own room. And it has a bannister to slide down. I like it a lot."

Is your home like Tommy's old one or like his new one? Perhaps it is still a different kind. There are many kinds of homes for families to grow in.

Each person, from the very beginning of his life, needs a very special "home" to grow in. Without the uterus in the mother's body, the fertilized egg cell would quickly die. The uterus provides everything needed—warmth, protection, food, and oxygen—for the 9 months it takes to grow into a baby ready to be born. During this time we say the mother is *pregnant.*

THE BABY GROWS

At first the baby-to-be is still so small the mother hardly knows it is there. It takes about 2 months before it starts to look much like a baby. By then it is about one inch long, and tiny arms and legs have formed. There is also a tiny head with eyes, ears, nose, and mouth.

After 4 months' time the growing baby is 5 to 6 inches long. It is now able to let its mother know that it is alive. She can feel it move its arms and legs. Mother is happy to know it is developing properly.

After this the baby grows more quickly. The uterus

stretches as it needs more room. The shape of the mother's body changes too. Many mothers-to-be wear fuller *maternity* clothes during the last few months of pregnancy.

After growing for 6 months, the baby looks much as it will when it is born. It is still only about 12 inches long. It is not ready to leave its warm room in the uterus yet. Its body is not able to breathe air or digest food. It will need another 3 months to grow.

Its lungs, stomach, and other organs develop while the baby grows chubbier. A little flesh on its bones will help to keep it warm when it leaves its mother's body. It doesn't sleep quite as much during its last 3 months in the uterus. Though it hasn't much space, it manages quite a bit of action. Baby takes daily exercises in kicking and wiggling.

After 9 months in the womb, babies are ready to live in the world. Some are born after only 7 or 8 months. These are called *premature* babies. They can grow to be strong and healthy. At the beginning of their lives, though, they need extra care. They are usually kept in *incubators,* which keep them warm and away from germs.

THE BABY IS SAFE

While the baby is growing in the uterus, it lies in a sac filled with liquid. It does not drown because it does not breathe

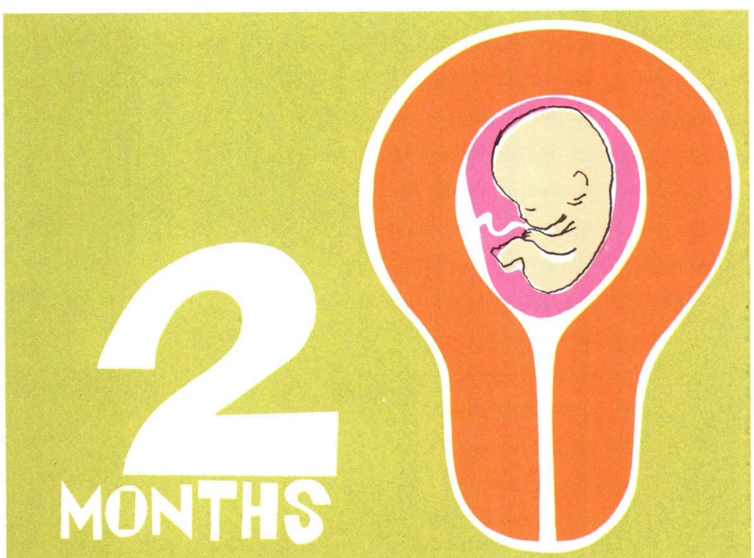

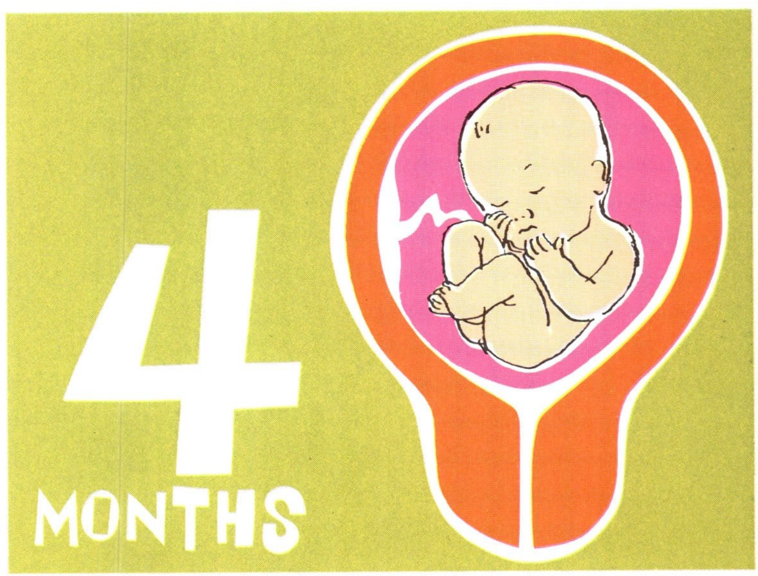

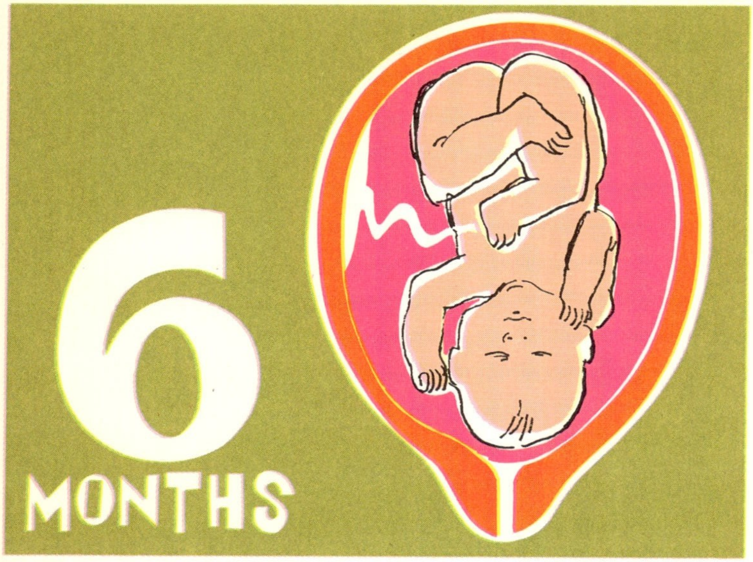

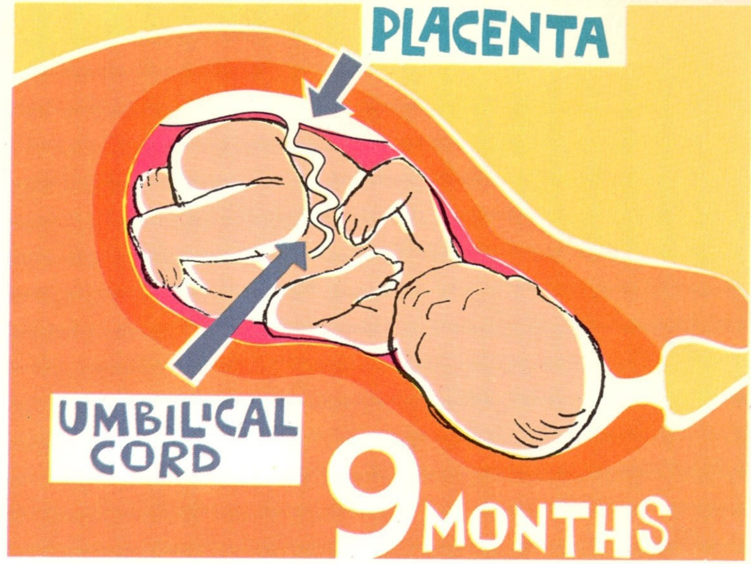

for itself yet. The water protects the delicate baby from being bumped or jolted in a way that could harm it.

Try this experiment to see how it works. Put a small ball inside a balloon, and fill the balloon with water. Now push your finger into the balloon from any side. You will find that the ball moves away from your finger. You may be able to tap the ball, but the cushion of water softens each bump.

THE BABY IS FED

The growing baby does not use its mouth for eating or its nose for breathing. Yet it gets all the food and oxygen it needs. Its mother's blood, which carries food and oxygen to all parts of her body, also brings both to the baby. The baby's food doesn't taste like steak or ice cream, for the mother has already digested it into simpler forms the baby can use. The food and oxygen pass from the mother's bloodstream to the baby's in the *placenta.*

The placenta is a network of blood vessels that grows on the uterus wall during pregnancy. In the placenta the mother's blood vessels lie next to the baby's. The mother's blood does not flow into the baby. Rather, the walls of the blood vessels act something like a screen or sieve. Food and oxygen move out of the mother's blood vessels into the baby's. The waste materials that collect in the baby's blood pass the other way, back into the mother's bloodstream. Her body then gets rid of them. The placenta also blocks the movement of larger germs from the mother to the child, thus protecting the baby from some sicknesses.

The baby's body is connected to the placenta by the *umbilical cord.* Through this cord the baby's blood carries food and oxygen to its body and waste materials away from its body. You can still see where this cord once joined your body. It is right in the middle of your abdomen. You may call it the belly button. A better name for it is the *navel.*

During the 9 months that a baby is growing in its mother's body the mother should eat good, nourishing food. Her health and the baby's depend on it, for she is actually "eating for two."

As the baby's birth comes closer, the mother also needs more rest. The other members of the family can help by being kind and considerate and helpful, so that she does not get overtired.

Everyone waits anxiously for the baby's birth. They enjoy guessing whether it will be a boy or a girl.

THE BABY IS BORN

When the time comes, the mother's body helps the baby to be born. For months the uterus has been stretching to give the baby room. Now it pulls together to push the baby out. The muscles of the uterus have to work hard to help the baby come

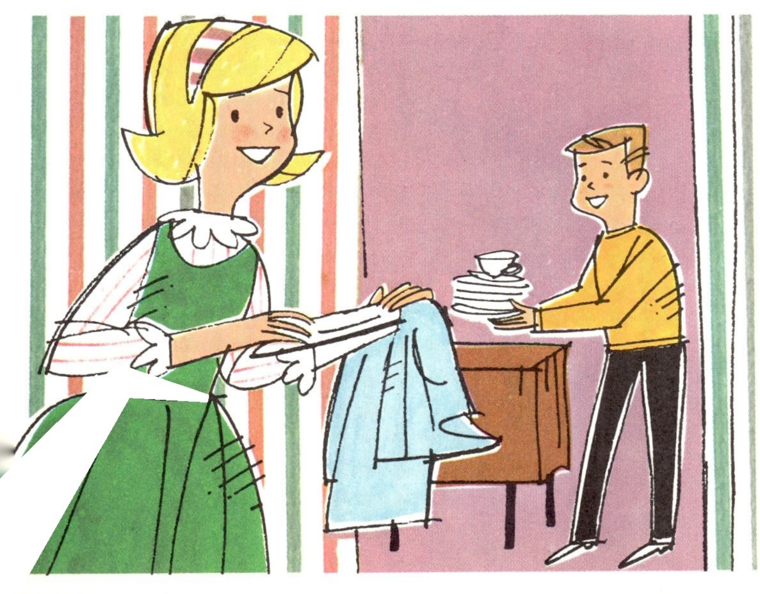

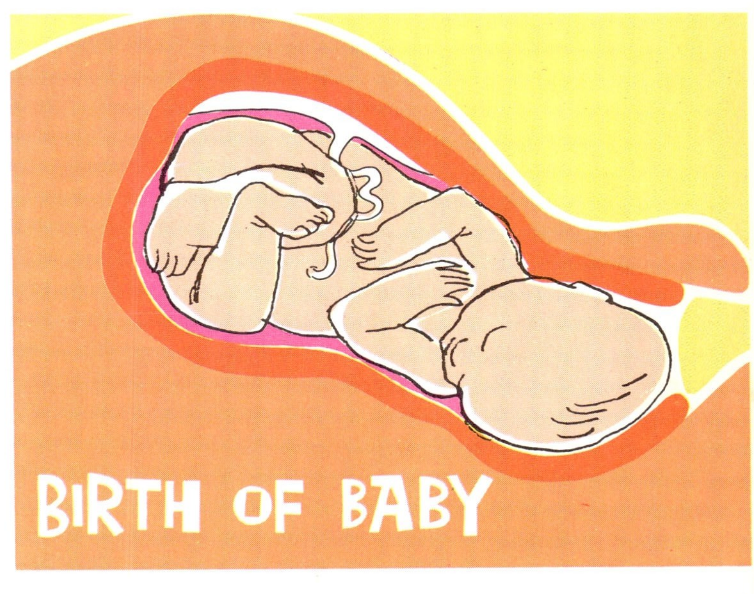

BIRTH OF BABY

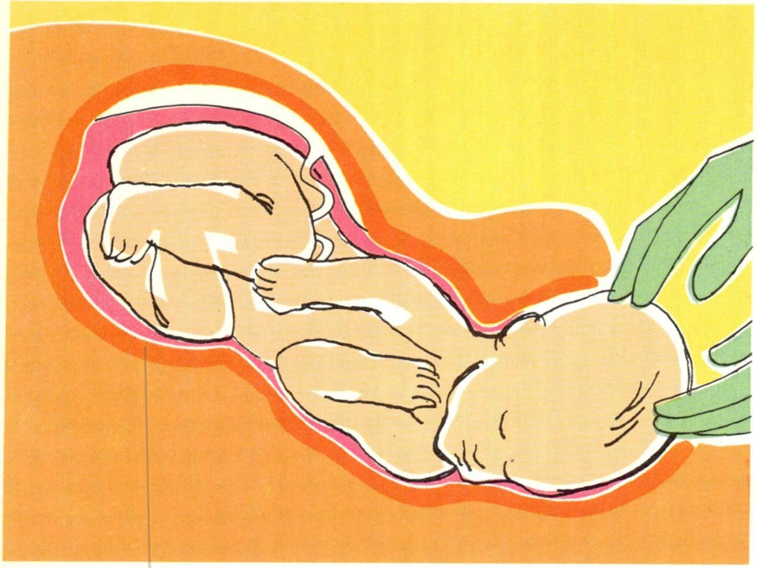

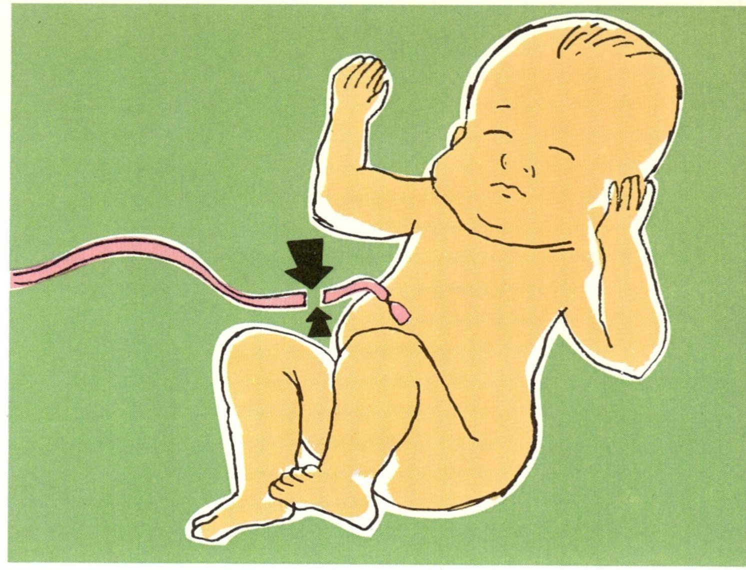

out. Mother usually goes to a hospital when this hard work, or *labor,* starts. There the doctors and nurses help the baby to be born. They take good care of both mother and baby.

During labor the muscles of the uterus push and rest, push and rest. The fluid-filled sac around the baby soon breaks. The baby is usually head down in the uterus, so the head comes first into the vagina, or birth canal. The vagina has to stretch, just as the uterus did, to make room for the baby. Soon the baby comes all the way out, usually headfirst. A nurse writes down the exact time it is born. This is an important moment.

The baby must breathe for itself now. It usually starts with a loud cry. Everyone is happy to hear a new baby cry. This means that it has started to use its own lungs and no longer needs to be attached to the placenta. Then the doctor ties and cuts the umbilical cord near the baby's body. It doesn't hurt either mother or baby, for there are no nerves in the cord. It is just like cutting your hair or fingernails, and will soon heal. The placenta, which is no longer needed, soon leaves the mother's body.

When the baby is born, the mother's breasts start providing milk to feed it. Milk is the only food the baby needs for a while. The newborn baby is pretty helpless, but it does know how to suck. At its mother's breast it takes the perfect food God

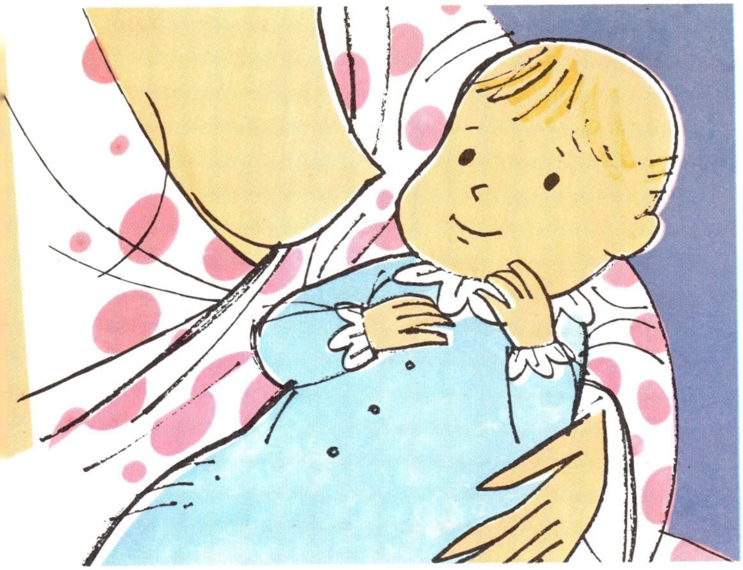

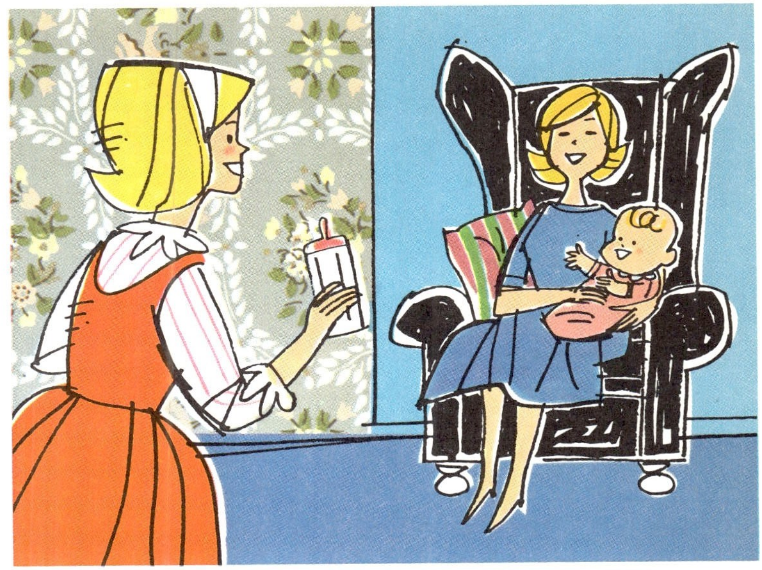

planned for babies. As mother holds baby close, it learns that it is loved and cared for.

A baby may also be fed with milk from a bottle. You have probably heard this milk called "formula." To make it much like mother's milk, vitamins, sugars, or water may be added according to the doctor's recipe or formula. Some babies may have particular needs that can be supplied only by a special formula. As mother feeds her baby from a bottle, she cuddles it lovingly.

AT HOME WITH THE FAMILY

A few days after baby's birth, mother and baby are ready to go home. But baby still needs care day and night. Father tries to help as much as he can. Children your age can help, too, by running errands, taking care of themselves, and keeping younger children happy.

Sometimes little brothers or sisters don't understand why people are so excited about a new baby. They don't know why the baby needs so much of mother's time and care. They may feel that mother loves the baby more than she loves them.

You know better by this time. A new baby needs more attention than the other children. Those who go to school can take care of themselves pretty well. They need only a little reminding, perhaps when it is time to take a bath or do homework. Smaller brothers and sisters can feed themselves, so even they don't need as much of mother's time as a newborn baby does.

A day has only 24 hours. You can't make a day longer by stopping the clock, can you? So all the children in a family have to share their parents' time. This may be difficult sometimes. But children who remember that their parents love them find it easier to share their attention.

When it is difficult for us to love others, it helps to remember that it may sometimes be hard for others to love us too. We are not always so lovable either.

But God showed us the way. He loved us enough to send Jesus into our world and into our lives. Through Jesus we become His children. In our baptism He made us members of His family. And now He continues to love us even when we are not so lovable. He forgives us and accepts us just as we are. And it is important for all members of a family who live together to do the same.

GIVE AND TAKE

Do you love your family? If someone asked you that question, you would probably answer, "Of course I do."

To answer the question, "How do you show your love?" you'd have to think a little longer. "Well," I hear you say, "there are six in my family. And they are all different. So I don't do the same things for each."

You are right. Each person is different and needs a different kind of love.

A baby needs to be cared for gently and tenderly. He needs cuddling often, but he can only smile in return. A child of 2 or 3 likes to sit on laps and have books read to him. He can show his love by welcome-home hugs and good-night kisses.

If you're a boy, perhaps you don't particularly like your mother to kiss you anymore—at least not when others are looking. You still love your mother, of course. You understand her better now. So you can show your love in more grown-up ways.

You can plan surprises that you know she will enjoy. You wouldn't do what one little girl did.

Five-year-old Janie once was taken shopping to buy a gift for her mother. Janie could think only of what she herself would like as a present. So she ended up buying her mother a doll. When Janie presented it, her mother had to smile at the strange gift. Mother knew how much her daughter still had to grow in her understanding and love.

Your love toward those in your family grows in this same way. Learning to know them better helps you do what will really please them. Understanding others makes us better able to appreciate the love behind their actions.

Learning to accept the love of others is important too. Giving and taking are both parts of a life of love. By offering love to others and accepting theirs in return, our love grows more like God's. He loves us and wants to be loved by us in return. Just so, we need to love and to be loved in return. This is what makes our life happy.

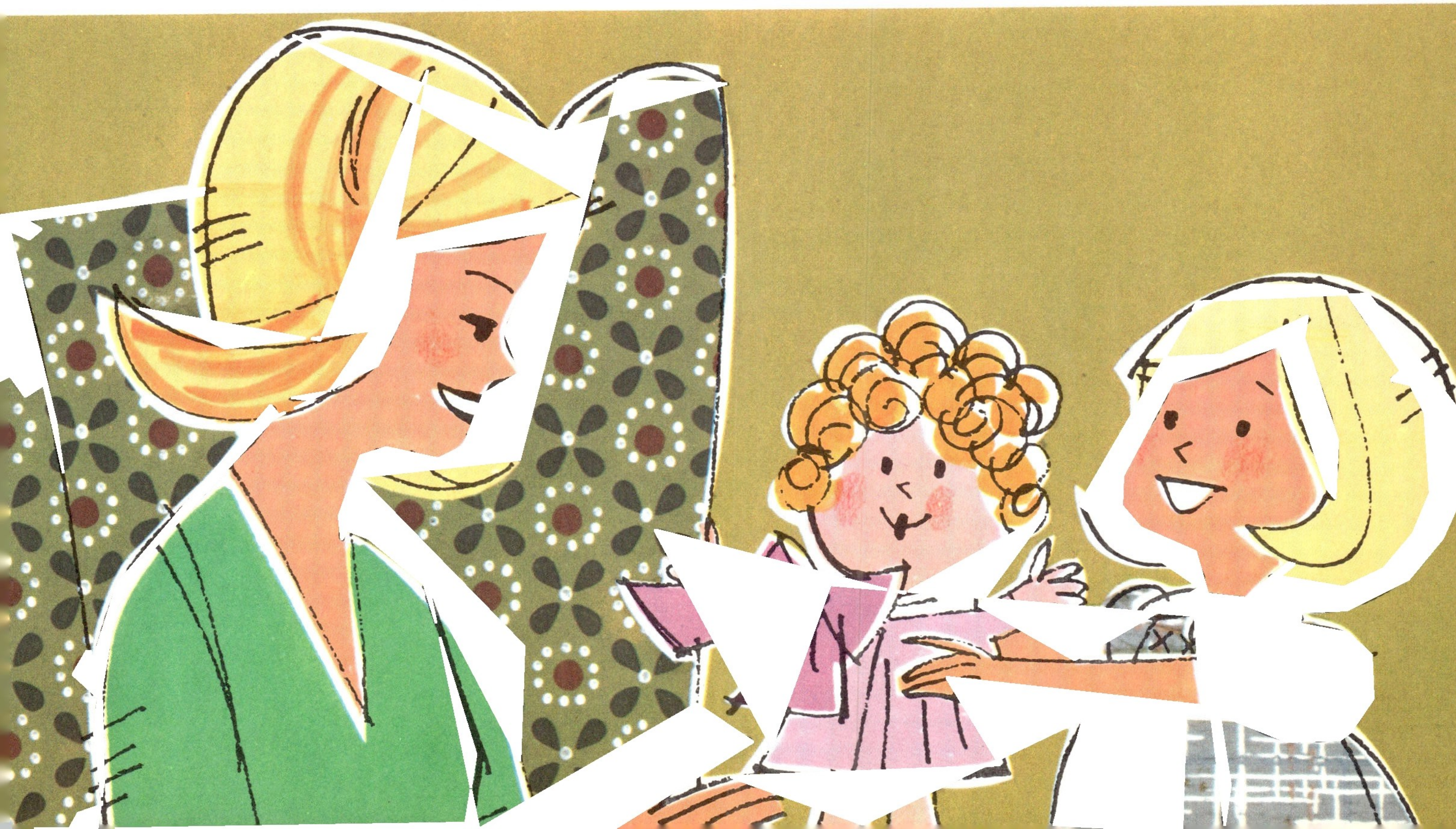

Where do you learn the most?

Most of us think of school when we think of learning. But it isn't all done there. The most important things we probably learn outside the classroom.

Whenever you are awake, you are learning. Long before you went to school, you were learning. In fact, your learning started as soon as you were born.

GROWING IS CHANGING

Some of the first things you learned were how to sit, stand, walk, feed yourself, and use the bathroom. You probably don't even remember that far back. But your parents do. They remember many things that happened as you used your five senses to explore and learn about the things and the people in this world.

They may have told you some of the mistakes you made as you learned. We all make mistakes as we grow up, but these stories may make you feel pretty silly now. Your father and mother remember them because they are interested in you and in your growing up.

As your muscles and nerves grew, you learned to do many things by watching others. Perhaps your parents took pictures of you at various times, as Ted's parents did. Ted was just one year old when he put Dad's big hat on his own little head.

His father and mother saved the picture because it was so funny. But it also shows how Ted was growing up. When Ted was born, he could not have done this even if he had tried, because his nerves and muscles were not yet ready.

YOUR CHANGING LANGUAGE

It also takes several years to learn to talk. By the time you were 4 months old, you already enjoyed hearing people talk. For many months you tried to make the sounds you heard.

Finally, when you were about a year old, you managed to say your first word. This was an exciting day for your father and mother. Perhaps they still remember your first "Da-da" or "Mama." Maybe they have it written down.

If you have ever listened to a small child, you know that we don't learn to talk all at once. Some sounds need lots of practice. Some words are too hard for little children. They may use easier or made-up ones. When going to the toilet, perhaps they say "wee-wee" or "big job." These expressions are probably a little different in each family. Such "baby talk" may not be understood by other people. That's why it is important to learn

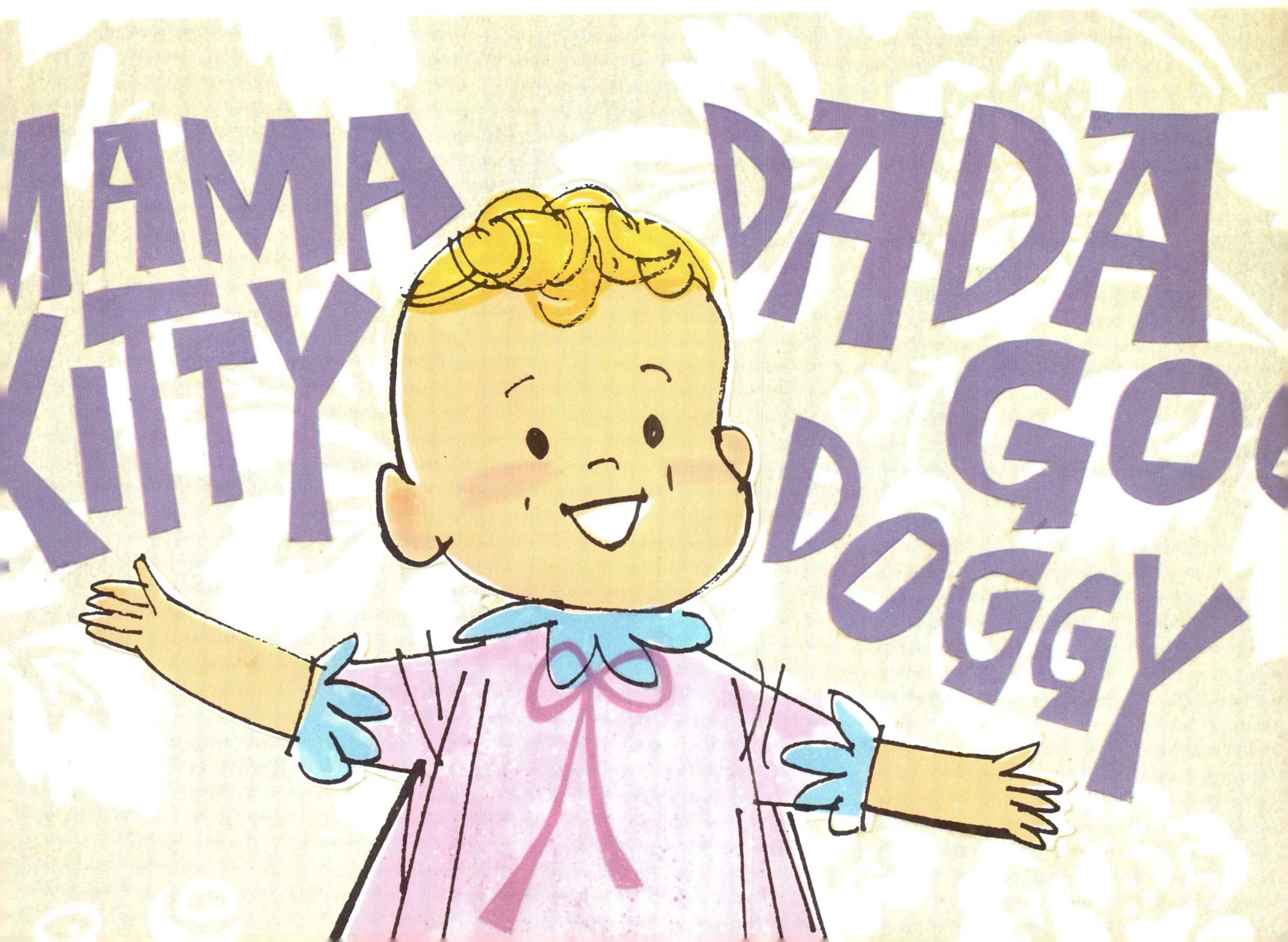

to use the proper words that everyone understands, like "urinate" or "bowel movement."

Don's father had helped him learn correct ways to speak of sex. But in the school washroom Don heard other things. He came home with a problem.

"Hey, Dad," he said. "Some of the kids at school use words that just don't sound decent. Why don't they use the correct ones?"

"Do they know them?" his father asked.

Donald had to think about that. "Maybe they never learned the right way to talk."

You have learned many of the correct words by reading this book. The list at the end of the book can make clear what each one means. Learning to use them correctly can be a big help in speaking of our bodies and sex in a grown-up way.

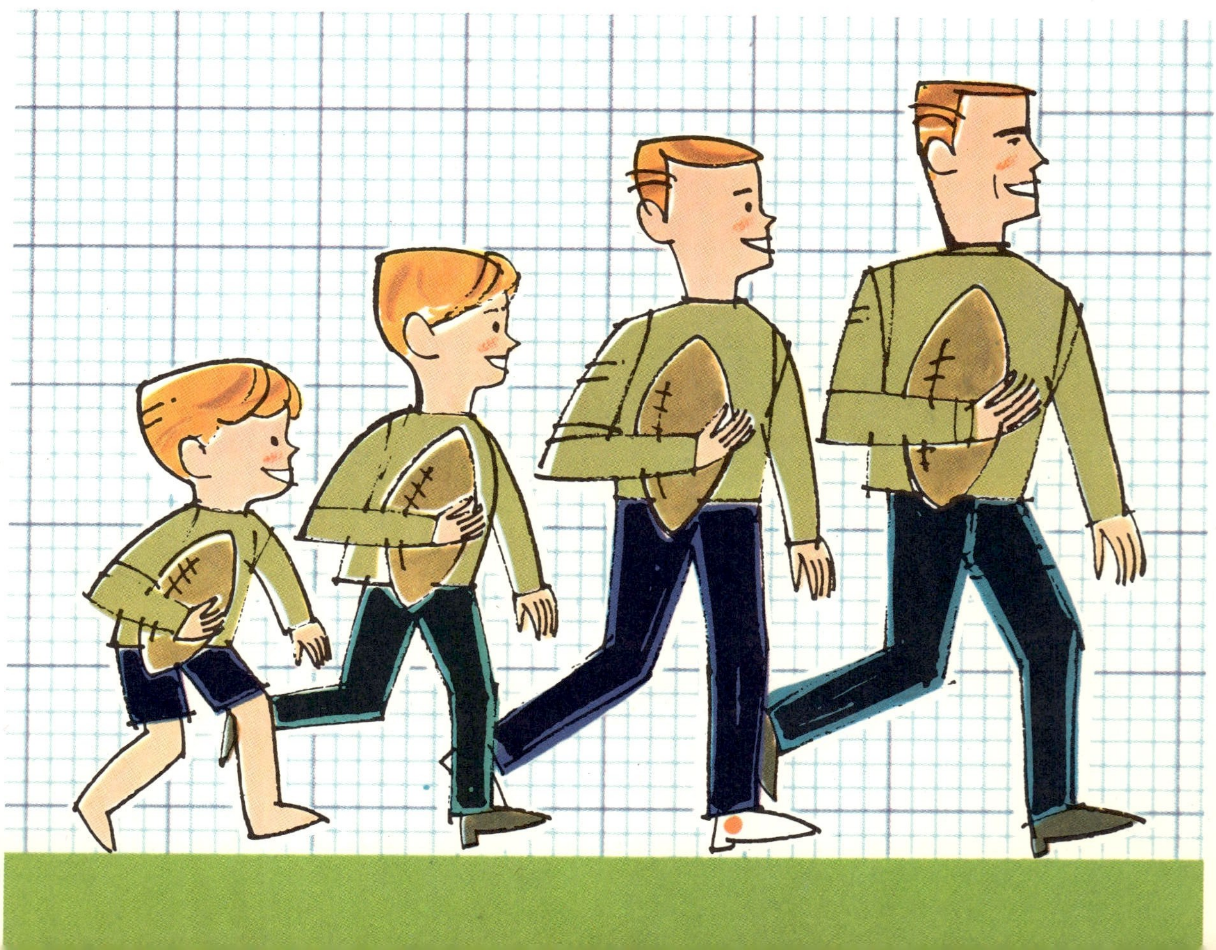

YOUR CHANGING FEELINGS

Just as our language becomes more grown up, so our feelings about our bodies change. The feelings a baby has about his body are different from the feelings an adult has. Babies like to explore their bodies. They may play with their toes, suck their thumbs, or handle their sex organs. It is perfectly natural for babies to do these things. How else can they learn about themselves?

By the time children are old enough to go to school, they have learned many things. They know the difference between boys and girls. But schoolchildren haven't learned all about their bodies yet. There are still many things they are puzzled about.

In the washroom at school, for example, boys may notice that the penises of some boys look different from theirs. There is a good reason for this. Some, for example, have been *circum-*

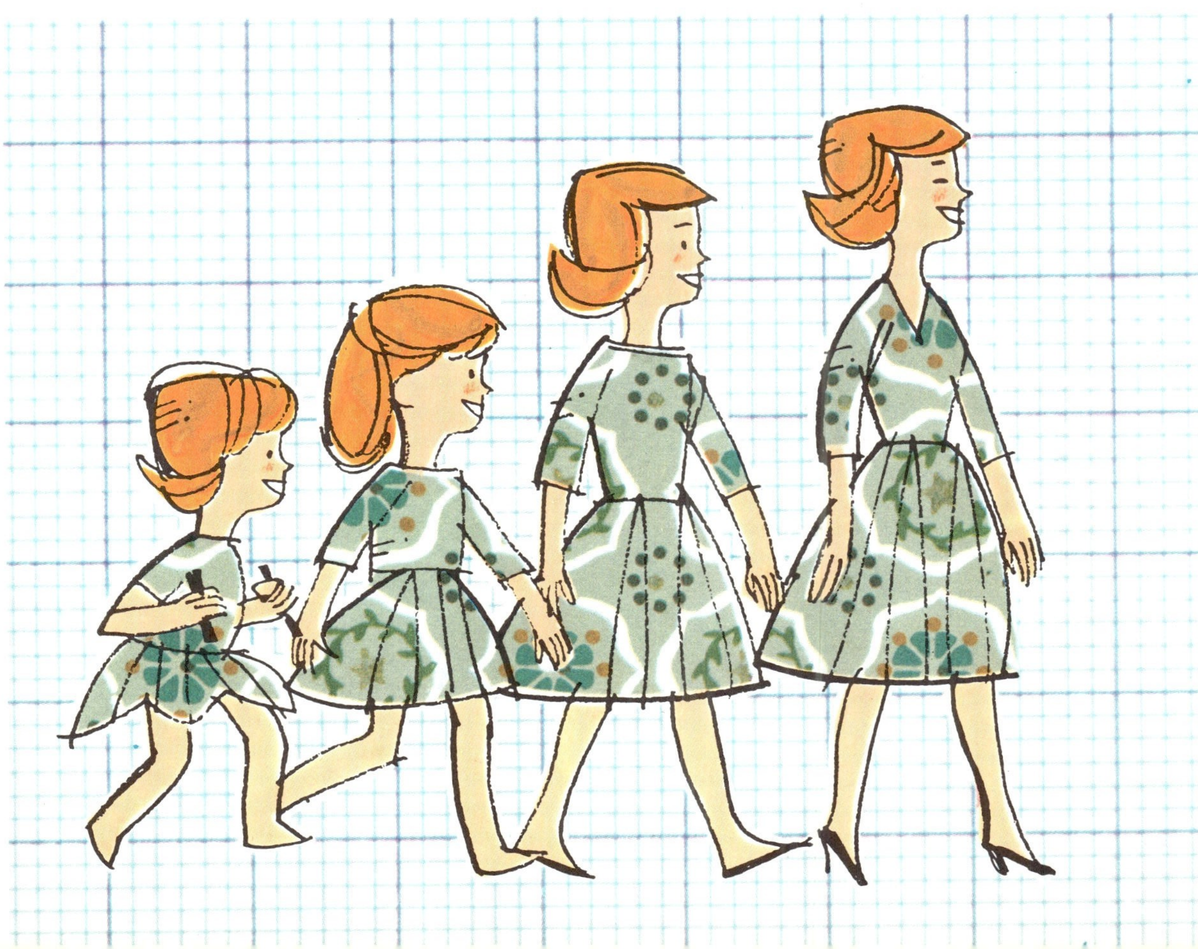

cised. When they were very young, the doctor cut off their *foreskin,* the loose fold of skin covering the end of the penis.

In Bible times God's people had their boy babies circumcised when they were about a week old. Joseph, for example, took Jesus to be circumcised on the eighth day after his birth. Even today most Jewish parents continue this Old Testament practice. So do parents who are not Jewish. But they do it mainly because doctors believe that circumcision aids good health. The penis is more easily kept clean when the foreskin has been removed.

Schoolchildren have questions about many things. There are many ways of learning the answers from reliable sources.

You should feel free to talk to your parents and teachers. Parents and teachers can help you understand many things you wonder about.

Some boys and girls your age may still play with their sex organs. They have a right to know about their bodies. But amusing themselves with such play is a babyish habit. People your age don't get fun out of fingering their toes or sucking their thumbs anymore. They outgrow such habits and find other things to do.

Some boys and girls may worry about doing such things. They may think that it is wrong. It isn't. Almost everyone does it when he is young. It isn't wrong. It's just babyish. When you have left such habits behind, you are on the way to being grown up.

YOUR CHANGING CUSTOMS

Little children have only good feelings about their bodies. They love to be free of their clothes. They don't mind if others see them bare. Two-year-old Joel was like that.

He had just finished his bath. His mother was patting him dry with a towel, but he wriggled away and ran down the hall. He laughed and squealed with delight. What fun it was to be bare. All those tight clothes were gone. His skin felt so warm and clean from his bath.

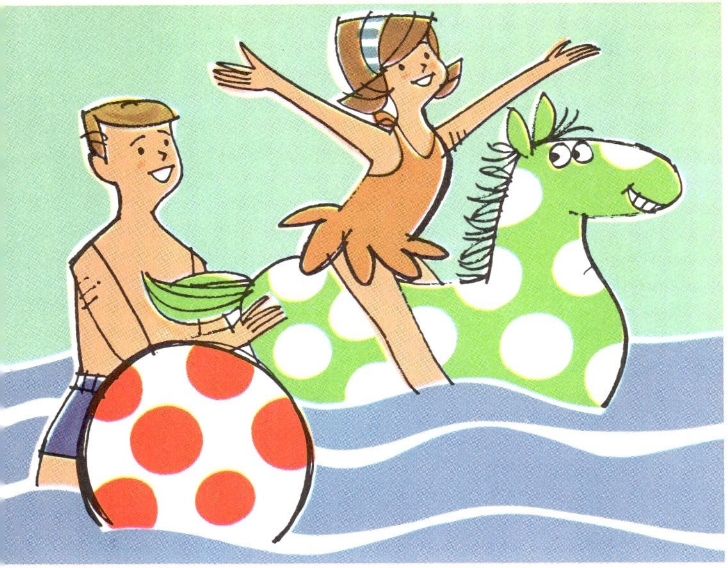

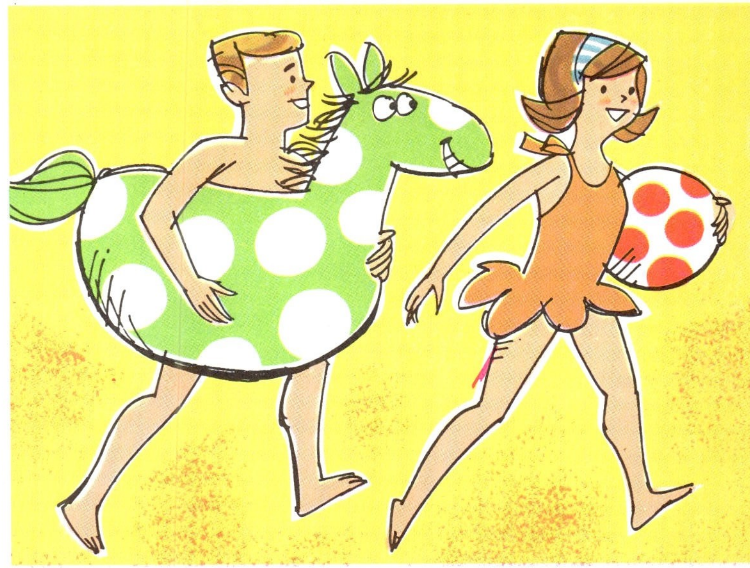

Your body feelings have probably changed since you were a baby. No doubt you have definite ideas about keeping your body covered. Most of these feelings you have learned from the rest of your family. Customs vary from home to home.

In some families everyone dresses and undresses in private. In others it doesn't matter where the children undress. Some families are used to having the door locked while someone is using the bathroom. In others the bathroom may be used by several at one time.

Some of your customs will probably change as you grow. There is nothing wrong with changing your mind about these things. You may, for example, take your bath alone now. In some high schools the girls take group showers, as do the boys. To some this seems natural. Others, who come from a school where there were individual showers may think it strange to bathe together.

Our customs may change, but our good feelings about our bodies should not. We have good reason to feel that our bodies are good. We were created by God.

A Christian feels proud of his body. For its creation he can thank God in words that men have used for thousands of years: "I will praise Thee, for I am fearfully and wonderfully made; marvelous are Thy works!" (Psalm 139:14). A Christian will give his body the best of care. He will use it as God wishes him to. He will respect it always.

IT'S GOOD TO BE ALIVE

"Alan, Alan," his mother moaned. "Why can't you ever hang your clothes up? And must you be so noisy?"

Sally's mother wasn't always satisfied either. "Sally, you used to be more tidy. Just look at your room! No wonder you are always stumbling over something."

Do these words sound familiar to you? People your age do have their problems and difficulties. No period of life is entirely without them.

But there is adventure, too, in your present life. There are so many interesting things to do, the days seem too short. Though your parents may not often tell you about it, they see your character developing as you take responsibility for your mistakes. As you learn to get along with those outside your family and find ways to be useful in your school and neighborhood, they see the promise of the man or woman you are becoming.

The time when you will grow up will be here sooner than you think. No, you won't turn into an adult overnight. It will take several years for the whole process to be completed. Many of the first changes are so gradual, they may take place without your realizing them.

The years of changing from a child to an adult are called *adolescence.* The teen-age years are often called by this name, though adolescence may start before age 13.

Teen-agers may seem grown up to you. Many boys and girls look forward to leading the life of a teen-ager. However, adolescence has its problems, as does any other time of life. Learning to be men and women is not always easy for boys and girls. Yet these years are full of exciting new experiences. So look forward to adolescence as a fascinating challenge!

ADOLESCENCE

One of the first signs of adolescence is a sudden spurt of faster growth. Most girls can expect it between 10 and 12; most boys, between 12 and 14. This period of more rapid growth may begin earlier or later. Some your age have already started to "shoot up." Perhaps you yourself have. Neither wishing nor worrying can change your growth pattern, for it is inherited. The foods you eat can influence your growth a little, but in a couple of years the late starters will usually catch up with the early birds.

What causes these two or three years of fast growth? How does the body know when to stop? There is much about the human body that is still a mystery. But we do know that *hormones* are a large part of the answer. They are the body's chemical messengers. They travel in the bloodstream, carrying

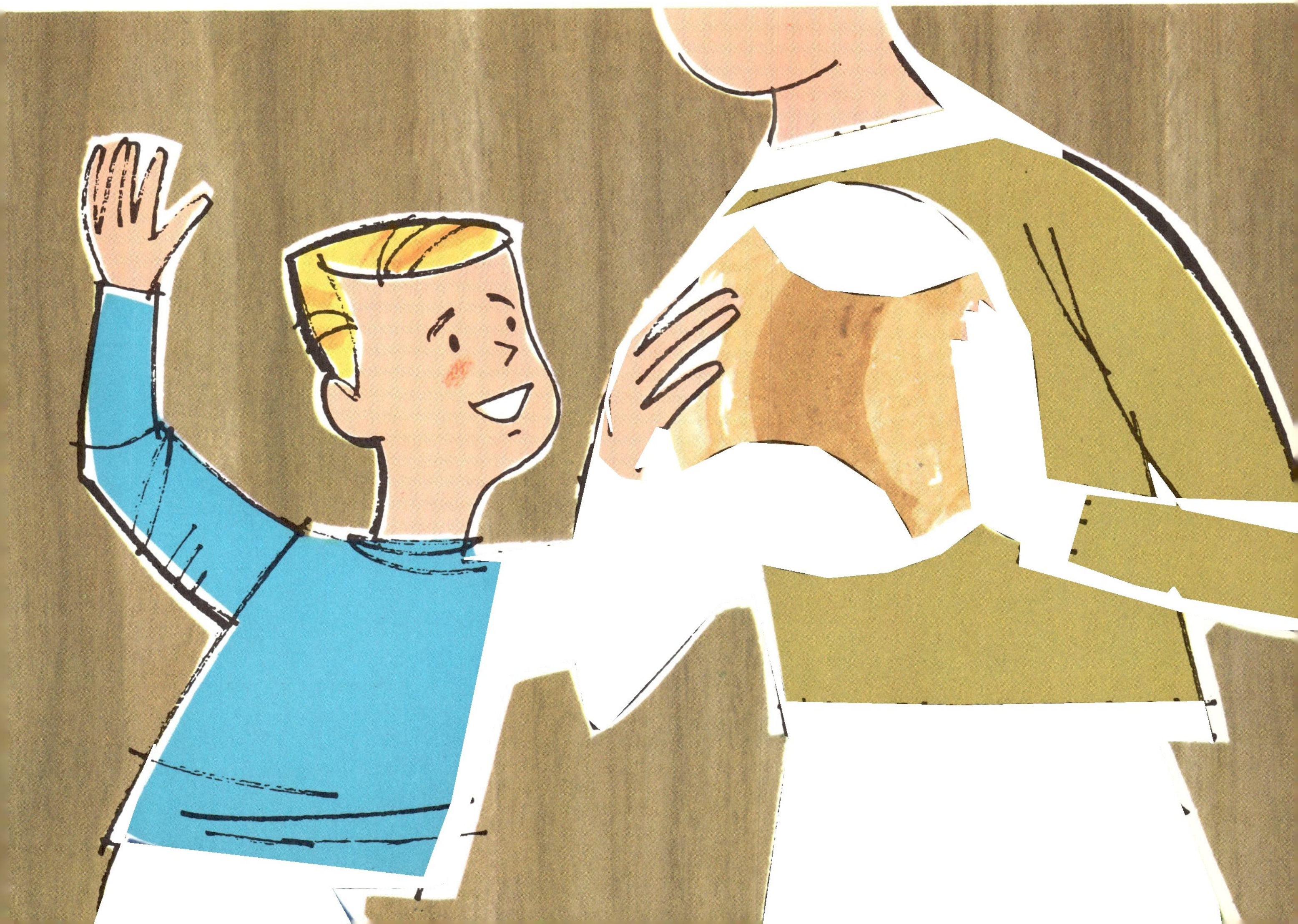

messages to various parts of the body. Each hormone signals a particular part of the body to start or stop an activity.

GIRLS

The ovaries of a girl produce hormones that make the growing-up period more than just a growing out of her clothes. A girl finds that, in addition to growing taller and gaining weight, the form of her body begins to change. Her breasts develop, and her hips become fuller. The straight lines of the little girl become the curves of the young woman. Hair starts to grow where none grew before, under the arms and on the lower part of the abdomen.

After a girl has been growing fast for a time, she is ready to slow down again. Just then a very sudden change takes place. Her ovaries begin to release mature egg cells. One of these eggs leaves an ovary each month. Each time this happens, the uterus gets ready to feed a fertilized egg cell. The lining of the uterus fills with an extra supply of blood. If the egg is not fertilized, it breaks apart and disappears. The extra blood in the lining of the uterus then leaves the body through the vagina. This is called *menstruation.*

Girls usually start to menstruate after their girlish figure has started to change to that of a young woman. Most girls are between 11 and 13. It is quite normal, though, to start anytime between 9 and 16.

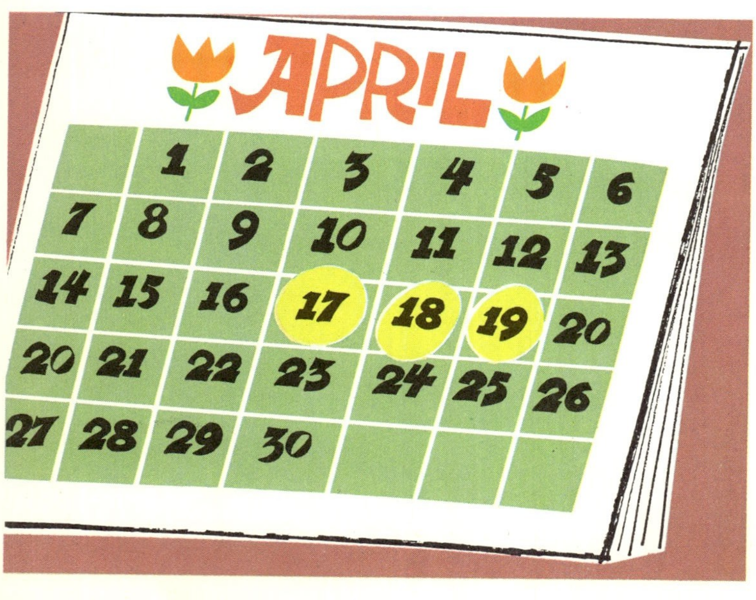

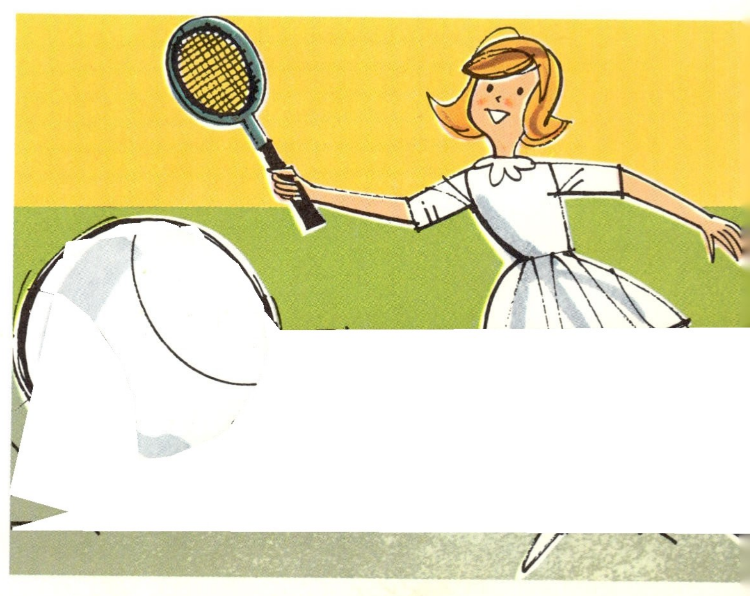

While girls are menstruating they wear sanitary napkins to protect their clothes. These pads are held in place by an elastic belt. Menstruation usually lasts from 3 to 5 days. Then the ovaries prepare to release another egg, and the same cycle starts over again. Since menstruation comes at regular times, it is often called a "period." However, young girls just starting may often skip a month or more.

Menstruation is a normal happening for women. It is good to continue most activities. Following the usual health rules will help a girl feel well during her period. It is particularly helpful to have good food and exercise and to take a daily warm bath.

When a girl starts to menstruate, she can have a new pride in herself. This is a sure sign that she is growing up and becoming a young woman. Her body is preparing for that day when she may become a mother.

BOYS

A boy's sudden spurt of fast growth comes usually around the ages of 12 to 14. A hormone gives the signal for growth to start and then to slow down again. It also sends a message to the boy's testicles. These sex glands produce the hormones that bring about the other body changes.

As the boy grows taller, he grows broader in his shoulders,

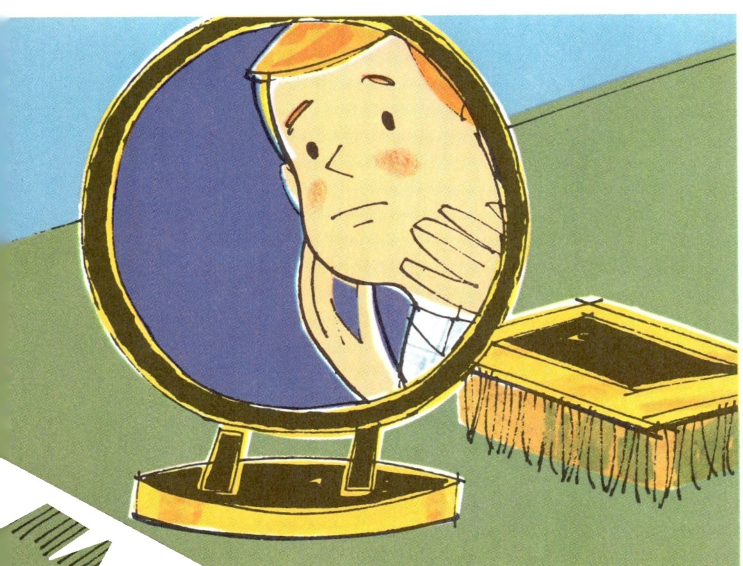

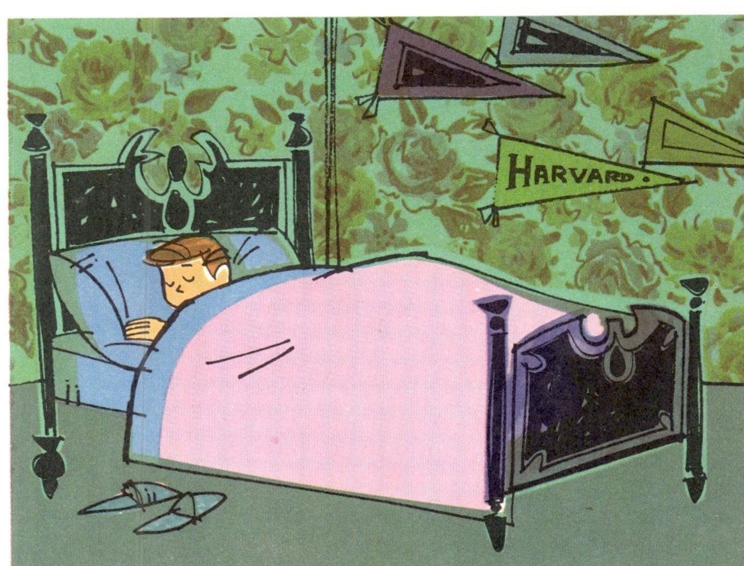

and his penis and testicles grow larger. His boyish voice changes to the deeper voice of a man. Hair grows on the lower part of his abdomen, under his arms, and maybe on his chest. The teen-age boy keeps a close watch for the first bristle to show on his chin. He can't wait to begin to shave like a man.

The testicles soon begin to produce sperm and store it up. During these adolescent years, the penis may at times become firm and erect, and semen may pass out of the body. These *seminal emissions* often happen at night during sleep. That is why they are called "wet dreams." They usually occur once or twice a month, but not as regularly as a girl's periods. They are a sure sign that a boy is growing up. His body is becoming a man's body, and someday he may be a father.

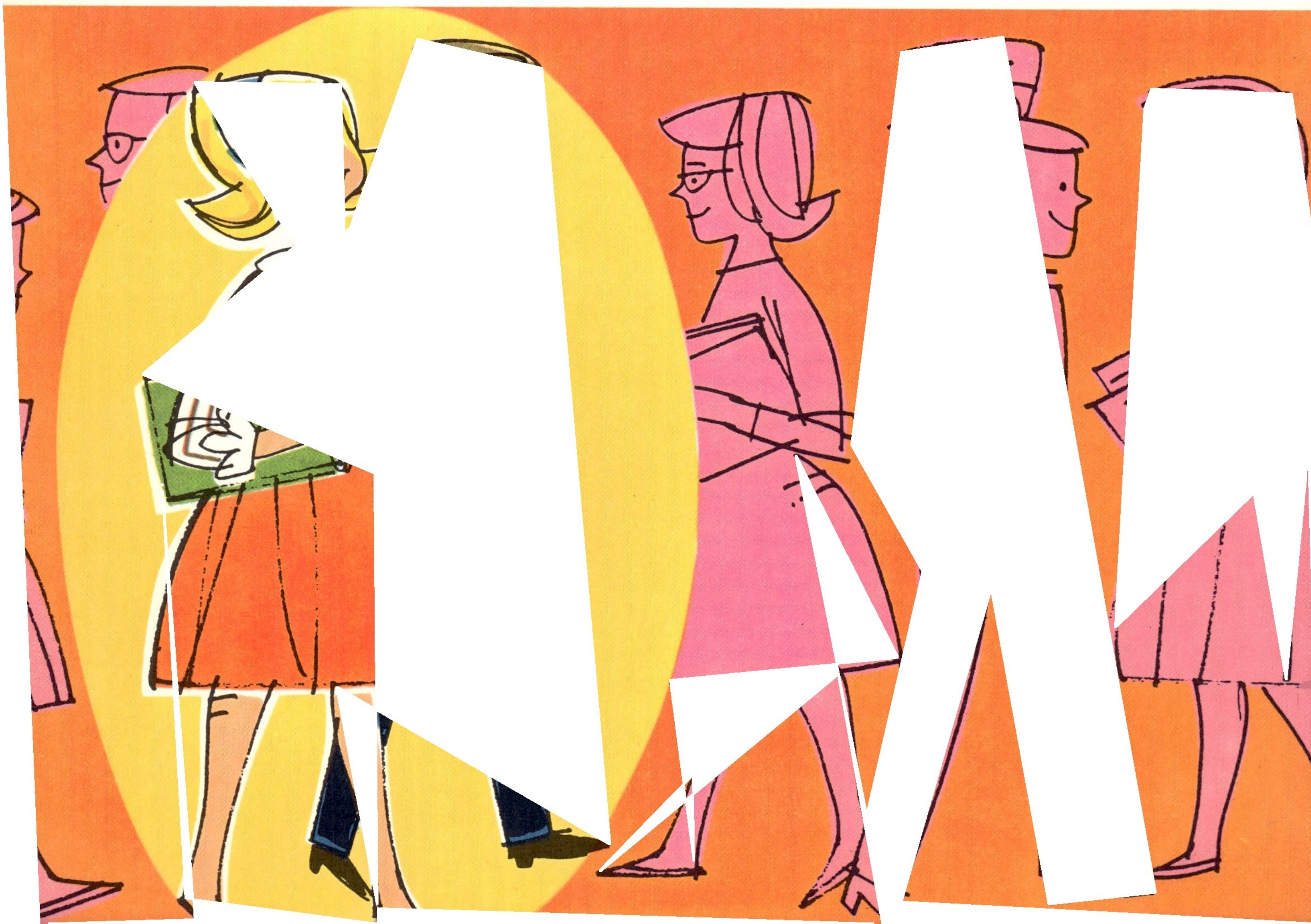

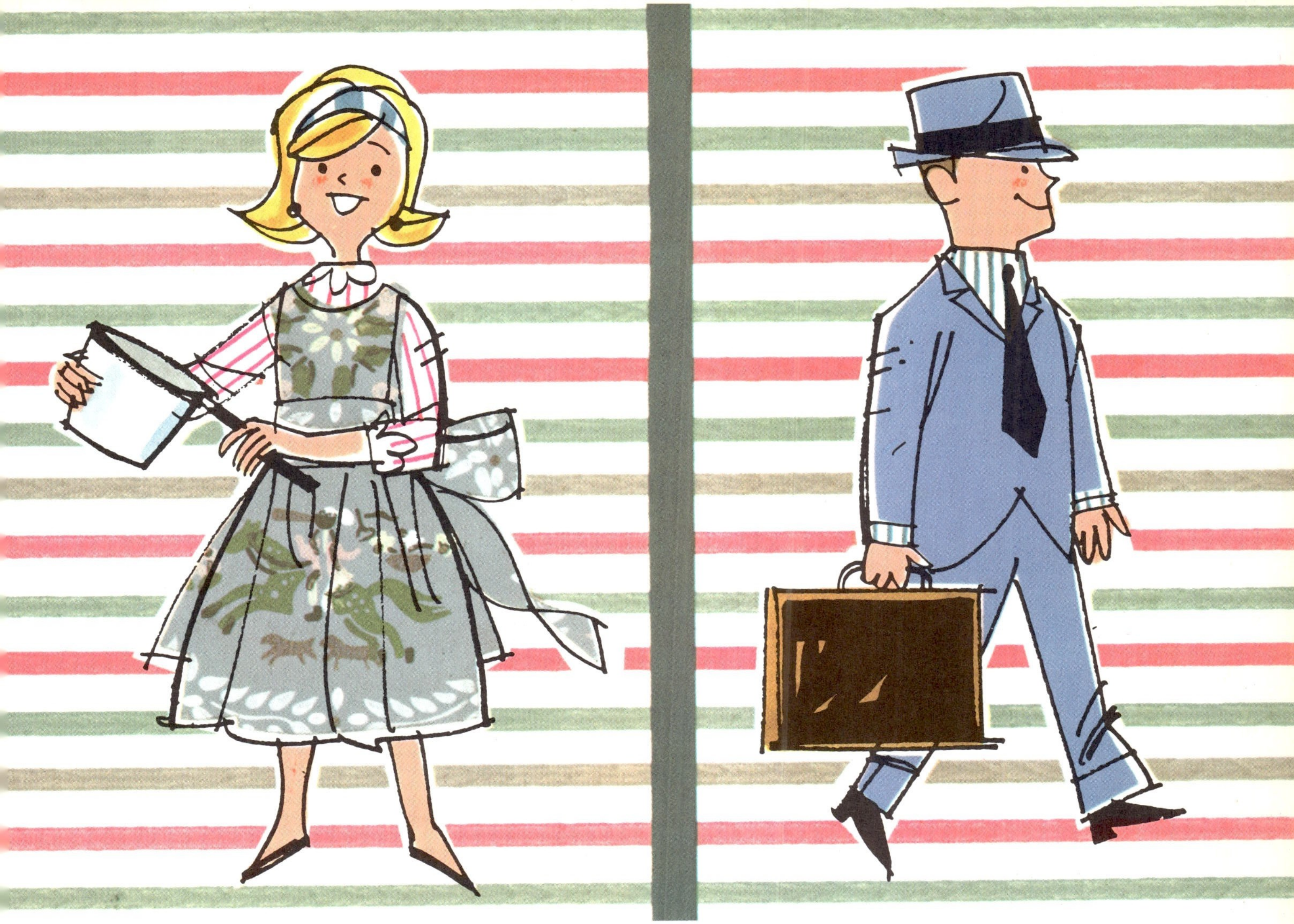

PREPARING FOR THE FUTURE

Thirteen-year-old girls may be able to produce egg cells. Their bodies can nourish a fertilized egg. Boys of 14 may be able to produce sperm. But these boys and girls are not yet ready to become mothers and fathers. There is more to being grown up than that.

Before boys are ready to get married and start a family, they must at least be able to earn a living. They must have a skill that will support themselves and their families. This means finishing high school. For many boys it means more—college or other job training.

Girls have many things to learn before they are ready to take a woman's place in the world. Besides learning homemaking skills at home or at school, many girls your age have learned something about child care. Helping with younger ones at home and baby-sitting jobs can give more valuable experience to future mothers. For girls too, finishing high school is extremely important, and college is advisable if possible.

The teen-age years are good years for making new friends and enjoying work and play with others the same age. A variety of friends help young people learn about many different kinds of people. In this way they decide which type of person they get along with best and which kind of friendship lasts the longest.

Knowing many different people will prepare you in deciding what kind of person you will eventually want to marry. Choosing a husband or wife is one of the most important decisions you will ever make. It will mean the difference between a happy home or an unhappy home in your future.

Your adolescent years will pass only too quickly. They will be full of experiences leading to adult life. During these exciting years, you will gradually start deciding for yourself the many things your parents now decide for you. As you make these decisions, you will need to remember who you are: a child of God and a Christian. Only then will you be able to discover God's will for your life.

God's will is that you remain His child, showing others in everything you do what God is really like. Because Christ loves you and lives in you, your life is bound to show it. God's love shining through you will become love and concern for others. Through a growing understanding of God's will, you can become more completely the person that you are.

For you have been wonderfully made. Your Creator expects great things from you. As part of His loving plan, He created your sex and all that goes with it. Because of this gift, you will one day have the privilege of working with Him in the creation of new life. As a father or a mother, you will be able to create a happy home for your children. By your love and care you will be able to show them a little of what God's love is like.

In the years to come you will be able to enrich the world in many ways. You are preparing for this future life even now, by growing up fully in mind and body, in feelings and abilities. At times you are beginning to taste the excitement of doing things for yourself and of making friends on your own. In times of difficulty, you realize the comfort of having a family to fall back on.

Difficulties will continue to come in the years of adventure ahead. It is good to remember that God is able to help whenever the growing or the going gets rough. When a mistake clouds your day or you just can't make it alone, He is there. With His forgiveness and help, you can start over and give life another try.

Jesus, your Brother, knows all about the problems that growing up brings. He was once your age, and He knows how it feels. Through His Spirit He is with you always. With His guidance you can decide for the right and the good in life. Following God's will always, you will be able to say, "It's good to be alive!"

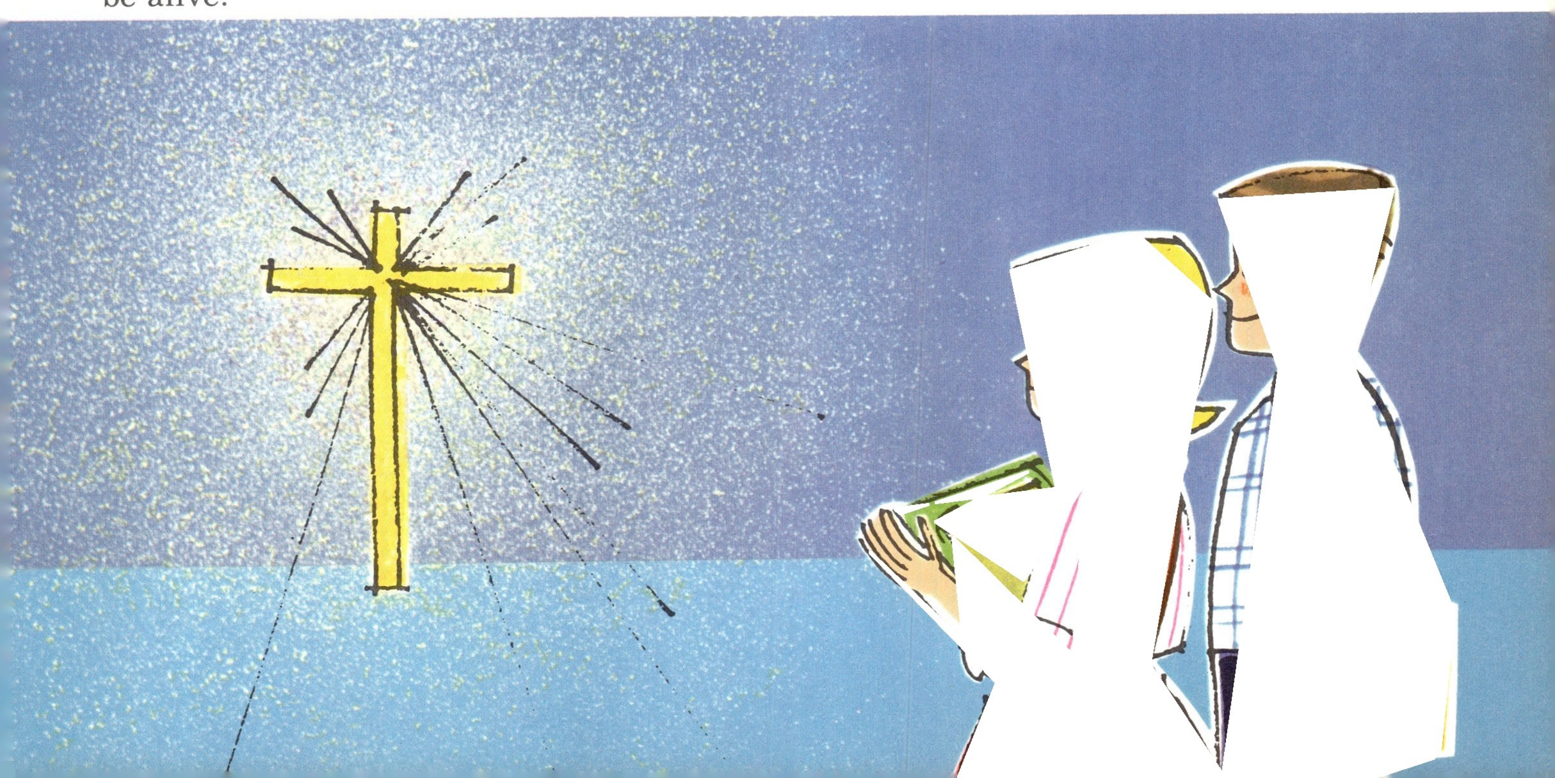

SOME WORDS USED IN THIS BOOK

abdomen (AB-duh-m'n; ab-DOH-men). The lower part of the trunk of the body; the belly.

adolescence (*ad*-uh-LES-'ns). The state, process, or period of life during which a child grows to adulthood; roughly, the teen years.

cartilage (KAHR-tih-lij). A firm, rubbery body substance that gradually converts and hardens into bone.

chromosome (KROH-muh-sohm). One of a usually definite number of small bodies, parts of which are genes, that are found in the cells of a given species.

circumcision (*ser*-kum-SIZH-un). A minor operation in which the loose skin, or foreskin, is removed from the end of the penis.

conceive (k'n-SEEV). To start a new life through union of a sperm cell with an egg cell; to become pregnant.

fertilize (FER-tuh-lyze). To make fertile, fruitful, productive, specifically by union of the male and the female reproductive cell to form a new individual; to make pregnant.

gene (JEEN). A small part of a chromosome that carries or determines an inherited trait.

genital (JEN-uh-t'l). Pertaining to reproduction or the organs of sex.

gland (GLAND). An organ that forms one or more substances to be used in, or eliminated from, the body.

heredity (hehr-ED-ih-tee). The sum of the qualities and characteristics passed on from ancestors to offspring.

hormone (HOR-mohn). A substance produced by a gland and carried by the bloodstream to stimulate and regulate the activity of other parts of the body.

identical (eye-DEN-tik-'l). Exactly alike or equal, as similar twins derived from a single fertilized egg.

incubator (IN-kyoo-*bay*-ter). A usually glassed-in bed or apparatus for special care of babies born early or sick.

labor (LAY-ber). The exertion and pangs of childbirth as a mother's body pushes to give birth to her baby.

maternity (muh-TER-nih-tee). The quality or state of being a mother; motherhood.

menstruation (*men*-stroo-AY-shun). The monthly flow of waste blood, secretions, and tissue from the uterus.

navel (NAY-v'l). The low spot or depression in the middle of the abdomen, marking the point from which the umbilical cord once ran to the placenta of the mother.

ovary (OH-vuh-ree). An almond-shaped female reproductive organ in which egg cells develop and sex hormones are produced.

oxygen (OKS-ih-jen). The most abundant element on earth, found free as a gas in the air, needed for respiration and life.

penis (PEE-niss). The male genital organ through which both urine and semen pass out of the body.

pituitary (pih-TYOO-ih-*ter*-ee). The body's master gland at the base of the brain. Its secretions control and regulate many other organs and thus influence most basic body functions.

placenta (pluh-SEN-tuh). A special network of blood vessels and tissue that develops on the lining of the uterus during pregnancy, to which the umbilical cord runs from the growing child and in which food, oxygen, and wastes are exchanged between mother and child without interflow of their blood.

pregnant (PREG-n'nt). Carrying a growing baby in the uterus.

premature (*pree*-muh-TYOOR). Too early, occurring before the proper time, as a baby born before the usual 9 months of pregnancy have passed.

reproductive (*ree*-proh-DUK-tiv). Relating to or used in producing again, as in the creation of new life.

scrotum (SKROH-t'm). The external sac of skin in which the testicles hang between the legs of a male.

semen (SEE-m'n). The male fertilizing fluid, composed of sperm and the whitish liquid in which they are suspended.

seminal emission (SEM-ih-n'l eh-MISH-'n). The discharge of semen from the penis.

sperm (SPERM). The male cell produced in the testicles for fertilizing the female egg.

testis (TESS-tis) or **testicle** (TESS-tik-k'l). The male reproductive gland in which sperm are produced.

uterus (YOO-ter-us). The hollow female organ for housing and feeding a baby during its development before birth.

vagina (vuh-JY-nuh). A passage leading from the uterus to the outside of the body; the birth canal.

virgin (VER-jin). A person—in usage usually female—who has never had sexual intercourse.

vulva (VUL-vuh). The external parts of the female genital organs.